MEDITERRANEAN DIET SECRETS

A QUICK START GUIDE TO HEALTHY, ANTI INFLAMMATORY FOOD FOR LONG-LASTING WEIGHT LOSS, WITH LIFESTYLE SECRETS, 70 DELICIOUS RECIPES, COOKBOOK AND EASY 14-DAY MEAL PLAN

LISA SCOTT

TABLE OF CONTENTS

Introduction..vii

   The Problem With Traditional Diets...ix

1: **What is the Mediterranean Diet?**..1

   Origins of the Diet..3

   Traditional Foods...4

2: **Why the Mediterranean Diet?**...11

   More Than a Fad..12

   No Deprivation and Reduced Cravings..16

3: **The Science behind the Mediterranean Diet**...................................19

4: **Secrets of the Mediterranean Lifestyle**...39

   Enjoy Fresh Food...41

   Spend More of your Income on food...43

   Choose Organic Food..44

   Next Steps..66

5: **Mediterranean Foods**...69

   Mediterranean Store Cupboard..69

   Food List...74

   Cut Back on These Foods..79

   Avoid These Foods...80

6: The Keto Mediterranean Diet 83

7: Ten Tips For Success 87

8: The 14-Day Mediterranean Diet   Menu Plan with Recipes 95

   Herbed Omelette with Spinach and Feta 100

   Spicy Chickpea Salad with Greens 101

   Crunchy Vegetable Wraps 101

   Instant Pot Mediterranean Chicken Casserole 102

   Strawberry Smoothie Cups 103

   Poached Eggs in Spicy Tomato Sauce 104

   Grilled Lemon Chicken with Parmesan Tomato 105

   Eggplant Parmesan 106

   Instant Pot Chocolate Pudding 108

   Blueberry Yogurt with Walnuts 109

   Steamed Vegetable Mix 109

   Caprese Salad 110

   Italian Hasselback Chicken 111

   Roasted Honeyed Almonds 112

   Italian Frittata with Cherry Tomatoes 113

   Avocado Salad with Smoked Salmon 114

   Tuscan Style Salmon 114

   Egg Stuffed Bell Pepper 115

   Shrimp and Summer Veggie Bowl 116

   Chili Roasted Chickpeas 117

   Skillet Chicken with Broccoli and Mushrooms 118

   Fig and Cherry Bites 119

   Berry Cinnamon Oats 120

   Cauliflower Pizza Crust 121

Sweet Potato Wedges 122

Cajun Chicken Lettuce Wraps 123

Raspberry Frozen Yogurt 124

Hash Brown Casserole 125

Lemon Parsley Pan Salmon 126

Parmesan Zucchini Sticks..127

Instant Pot Stuffed Chicken..128

Strawberry Cheesecake 129

Tuscan Mini Quiche...130

Crispy Feta with Eggplant Ribbons 130

Instant Pot Savoury Cauliflower Fritters...132

Seafood Stew 133

Greek Yogurt Chocolate Mousse...134

Breakfast Avocado Salad 134

Arugula Salad with Pine Nuts and Feta 135

Creamy Chili Shrimp 136

Coconut Cashew Bars 137

Baked Eggs with Tomatoes, Olives and Feta 138

Balsamic Glazed Caprese Chicken 139

Mediterranean Stuffed Peppers 140

Sweet Peppercorn Salmon 141

No Bake Fruit Tart 142

Fruit and Nut Yogurt 143

Tomato Cucumber Salad with Feta and Olives 143

Stuffed Zucchini Boats 144

Poached Pears with Walnuts...145

Zucchini and Tomato Frittata..146

Grilled Chicken Skewers 147

Strawberry Smoothie 148

Eggplant Hasselback 148

Cashew Cream Stuffed Strawberries 149

Egg White Scramble with Spinach and Tomato 150

Avocado Cucumber Chickpea Salad 151

Caprese Style Portobellos 152

Tuscan Skillet Chicken 153

Goats Cheese and Pistachio Stuffed Figs 155

Crumbly Berry Breakfast Bake...155

Crispy Parmesan Chicken with Vegetables 156

Herb Roasted Red Potatoes 157

Garlic Lemon Salmon 158

Apricot Energy Bites 159

Bonus Instant Pot Recipes 160

Instant Pot Chicken in Red Wine Sauce...160

Instant Pot Margherita Casserole 161

Mediterranean Hummus Recipe 162

Ratatouille (4 servings) 163

Coq au Vin (Chicken in Wine) for 4 people 165

9: Afterword 167

10: One More Thing..169

INTRODUCTION

What if you could find a diet, that was easy to follow, helped you lose weight and tasted great?

What if that diet also helped you to live better, for longer?

Sounds too good to be true, right?

The Mediterranean diet is not about counting calories.   In fact, the Mediterranean diet is not really a diet at all – it's a lifestyle.

It's all about the food you eat, what physical activities you participate in, and how you socialize with family and friends.

Most restrictive diets aim to act as quick fixes. They promise to deliver results, fast.

INTRODUCTION

Sometimes these diets work but, more often than not, it's just a temporary fix. You end up reverting back to the old ways, eating the wrong types of foods and gaining the weight right back again.

The Mediterranean diet is about making a real change to your life. It's about preventing disease and decay. It's a way of life, that can reduce your chance of diseases such as cancer, heart disease and diabetes.

Remember how good it feels when you go on vacation in the sunshine? It's great to eat fabulous food, relax and enjoy life. You return home feels refreshed and rested, with your body feeling vibrant and alive.

What if you could incorporate some of this feeling into your everyday life? What if you could eat delicious meals, take time to relax and regularly enjoy spending time out in nature or with family and friends?

Do you think that would make a difference to how you feel? Do you think that your body and mind would benefit from the change in your diet and lifestyle?

Of course they would!

So many diets take just one aspect of our life, such as diet or exercise, and suggest that changing a single aspect can impact your life.

The Mediterranean diet is different. It's a holistic approach, which focuses on the whole person, rather than any one aspect of your life.

The Mediterranean diet is a lifestyle, that focuses on more than just what you eat. It's about taking life one step at a time, embracing community, being more mindful and involved with what you eat.

It's a diet that can give you more life in your years, keeping you mentally and physically active for longer.

It's about a new way of living, about developing new healthier habits that can last a lifetime. It's about eating great-tasting foods that make you feel vibrant and alive.

Let's compare that, for a moment, with the traditional diets you might have tried in the past.

The Problem With Traditional Diets

Our society seems to have the idea that things are designed to be used up, thrown away, then replaced.

There's a focus on speed, on how something can be quickly achieved, with little emphasis on taking the time to enjoy life.

We all want to live a fulfilling life, we may even know what it takes, but few of us have the patience it takes to really find discipline in our lives to do what's needed.

We might choose the solution of quick diet pills, extreme exercise, or "cleanses", some of which come with unpleasant side-effects. These things can work, but only for a short time.

Most diets offer a short, sharp fix, but don't do anything to change the underlying problem, that is, your unhealthy lifestyle and diet.

The reason why so many of us find that we can't lose weight or keep the pounds off, is because we're expecting that quick fix. We're not willing to give any long-term commitment that might make a real difference to our life.

INTRODUCTION

In order to live a healthier life, it's more than just about the food you eat. There needs to be a real shift in the way you go about your day-to-day life.

Most of us are living life at a breakneck speed, feeling stressed and out-of-control.

The impact of modern living has made us feel as if we can't do anything to change the way we live.

We work 9 to 5 jobs, go home and do the chores, only to have to go to sleep feeling tired and wake up early the next morning, only to do it all again.

We find ourselves trapped in an unhappy cycle. It can feel as if we just don't have the time to make any change to our lives. We certainly don't have time to follow yet another diet!

It might seem like you have to go to the gym every night, try the latest diets and buy a bunch of new cookbooks in order to see the results you want.

But there is a solution, a way of the merry-go-round of life and it's much simpler than you might imagine: it's called the Mediterranean diet.

The Mediterranean diet is easy to maintain. It can fill you with energy, helps you lose weight and is great for your health and wellbeing.

If you follow the Mediterranean diet and lifestyle, you won't have to worry about crazy side-effects from your diet. You won't have to worry about gaining back all that weight you lost.

Eating healthy foods will become a habit, something you barely even think about.

Unlike some other diets, there's nothing extreme about the Mediterranean diet. No fad dieting, no crazy exercising, just a sustainable, enjoyable life, that you'll learn to love.

All you need is a desire to change or a passion for finding a better lifestyle.

The Mediterranean diet has been proven over decades, by millions of people. It works. It's a long term solution to your health and weight issues, rather than a quick fix.

It's not something a doctor has created, but something that scientists discovered, after looking at the lives of real people.

After a few days on the Mediterranean diet, you'll start to feel much better. Your digestion will regulate, your breathing will get easier, and you'll feel much better in general.

You might not look in the mirror after a week and see a dramatic weight loss; but let's get real, is there really a diet that's actually going to do that for you long-term?

The Mediterranean diet can produce permanent weight loss, but it's not going to happen overnight. It can help you maintain your weight too, something few diets actually address.

It's a diet that's not only filling, but also tastes delicious. When it tastes this good, it makes it easy to maintain your diet. In fact, you'll probably forget you're on a diet at all.

You aren't even going to feel hungry. We've become used to the idea that dieting about feeling permanently hungry. We can feel anxious, thinking that we'll have to give up the foods we like, or feel hungry, in order to see the results we want.

The Mediterranean diet is filled with foods that are rich and filling, so you never have to worry about going hungry.

INTRODUCTION

If you love to snack, this diet will be right up your street. Snacking is actually encouraged in a Mediterranean diet. You can snack on nuts, seeds, and fruits. Multiple small meals a day help keep the metabolism running, often producing a higher weight loss.

The Mediterranean diet means that you don't have to give up eating foods that taste great. Instead, your goal is to make more conscious choices and decisions for your health, not for convenience.

The Mediterranean diet doesn't feel like just a diet. It's a change of lifestyle. It's not another book to read and follow for a few weeks, it's a way of life that can help you feel more vibrant, prevent common diseases and prolong your life expectancy.

Many popular diets leave people hungry, hopeless, and disappointed. That's why they're called 'fad' diets - they come and go, because they're simply not workable and require a strict, disciplined food or exercise regime.

The Mediterranean diet is all-inclusive. Anyone can participate, and it doesn't take anything but a willingness to try new things. It's a diet that the whole family can eat - no more cooking one thing for them and another for you.

The best way to get started with a Mediterranean diet is to include family members, if you can. With your family on board with your healthy lifestyle, it's more likely there will be a positive outcome.

Having a support system that you can depend on really comes in handy, especially when experiencing a significant change in your lifestyle.

Eating healthily with others, can help prevent you sliding back into your old ways, getting fast food and sitting in front of the television while you eat.

Like any change in your life, the Mediterranean diet may not be easy at first, it'll probably take some work to make the changes; but eventually, it will become an easy and enjoyable way of life.

The Mediterranean diet is something that you can live on for life, without ever having to feel deprived. For those people living around the Mediterranean, it's their way of life.

Please note, I am not a professional nutritionist or someone with a medical degree. Any changes you make to your life, you are responsible for. When going through any significant diet and lifestyle changes, it is always best to consult a physician to ensure there won't be any health risks.

Although the Mediterranean diet is low-risk, it's still best to seek professional medical care to ensure this is the right diet for you.

I know, from personal experience, that following the Mediterranean diet can drastically help a person lose weight, maintain that weight loss, and be a much happier person overall. That's what's so great about the Mediterranean diet.

Whether you are vegan, vegetarian, or pescatarian, or have other dietary restrictions, the Mediterranean diet can work for you.

Don't worry, if the thought of eating olives or hummus scares you off, there are plenty of other foods you can enjoy!

Once you've read this book, you'll be ready to embark on your journey towards a healthy Mediterranean life.

Over the next few chapters you'll:

- have a comprehensive understanding of what the Mediterranean diet is

- understand some of the science and health benefits behind it

- know what foods can be eaten and which foods to cut down on or avoid

- be able to check out quick-start 14-day meal plan, complete with recipes

- discover how to embrace the Mediterranean diet and lifestyle for life

If you're up for the challenge of living a new, healthier way that will give you energy, help you stay healthy and lose weight, then read on!

1

WHAT IS THE MEDITERRANEAN DIET?

The Mediterranean diet is all about simple cuisine. It's about a diet and lifestyle, one that's enjoyed by the nations that live on or around the Mediterranean Sea.

It's a traditional diet, that's evolved over thousands of years. It reflects what was originally the 'poor mans' diet - eating those foods that locals were able to grow or catch locally, and adding fresh herbs to enrich the flavor.

The typical Mediterranean diet is abundant in fruits, vegetables, bread, other forms of cereals, potatoes, beans, nuts, and seeds.

The diet includes olive oil as an important fat source, with fish and poultry consumed in low to moderate amounts, and eggs and red meat consumed in moderation. You'll be pleased to learn that moderate intake of wine is also part of this diet.

On the Mediterranean diet, you'll cut out processed or convenience foods and enjoy cooking tasty meals from scratch. When you start with delicious ingredients, it's easier than you think to create great meals that you'll love to eat.

It's a diet that's about how you live your life. Of course, what you eat is important, but so is our pace of life and the relationships we have with those around us. Our stress and disconnected lives can be unhealthier for us than we imagine.

People living around the Mediterranean seem to know something about having healthy relationships. They have clear lines between work and home life, so don't have the same problems relaxing that people in western cultures do.

They're intentional about living life the way it's supposed to be. They take time to enjoy life, without allowing the stress from work to interfere. They put a real emphasis on family and community.

Many cultures have diets that revolve around where they live. People in tropical areas will likely have diets high in fish and fruit. Those that live in colder or landlocked areas might eat heavier foods that fill them up or rely on red meat as a source of protein.

Those that live in the Mediterranean have access to fresh food, fish, and fresh, local produce.

But you don't have to actually live near the Mediterranean to eat like the Greek, Italian or French do. Everything you need to live a Mediterranean lifestyle can be found on your grocery stores shelves.

Not everything will be exactly as it might be in Greece or Italy, of course. The foods won't be exactly the same, but what's more important is following the traditional ideologies that those who are on a Mediterranean diet follow. By doing this, you can begin to experience the quality of life that those in the Mediterranean enjoy.

Let's delve a little bit deeper into the history of the Mediterranean diet. When you understand something of their history, you'll see that this is much more than just a fad diet.

The Mediterranean diet follows a lifestyle that has come naturally to many people of the Mediterranean.

The French, Greeks and Italians haven't studied the optimal way to eat or cook food. Instead, it comes naturally to them, based on the resources that surround their homes and their shared love of great-tasting food.

Origins of the Diet

The diet itself is based around that of the people of the Mediterranean, which is where the name comes from.

The Mediterranean diet and lifestyle goes all the way back to Greek and Roman times, when the people of these cultures would snack on wine, cheese, and bread all throughout the day.

It's typically associated with French, Greek or Italian culture, as well as some of the other countries which border the Mediterranean Sea.

It all started back in the 1960's, when scientists discovered that the people living in Crete had a much higher quality of life. Crete is an island in the Mediterranean, and is part of Greece.

The scientists noticed that their overall health was improved, and that Cretans would often live longer than those in western cultures. As the results of the study became more widely known, people around the world started adopting the Mediterranean diet and lifestyle.

It's not just the food you eat that makes a difference, it's also how you live your life. That's one of the things that they do differently around the shores of the Mediterranean.

If you were to stroll down a typical French, Italian or Greek street and observe people, you'd notice several things about them. They're not in a hurry. They stop and talk to their neighbors, or the cashiers in the local stores.

Many of the locals have a small vegetable plot where they take pride in growing their own herbs and vegetables.

When they eat, they eat leisurely, savoring the tastes, not rushing their meal. More often than not, they'll eat with friends or family, rather than eating alone.

They're physically active - not the kind that you get from going to the gym, but the kind that you get by doing something meaningful, such as gardening, going out fishing, or walking to the local store.

They work hard and they play hard - at the weekend, the beach or the seaside restaurants are filled to bursting, with everyone unwinding and enjoying themselves.

Living around the Mediterranean means that there's plenty of sunshine. Constant sun exposure means increased levels of vitamin D, which can help prevent inflammation, something which is at the root of many of today's diseases and illnesses.

Traditional Foods

There are several foods that are important when creating a Mediterranean diet plan.

As you read on, remember that this diet is different from any other. One thing that surprises many users is that bread is allowed in the diet and is actually encouraged.

Many diets, especially those that are low-carb in nature, put a focus on eliminating any and all bread. Many people go to great lengths to avoid bread and any carbohydrates in general, believing that these carbohydrates will eventually turn into fat cells.

Those that eat Mediterranean know that when they eat whole grain breads, their body can use this as an energy source rather than fat storage. Of course, it's important to everything in moderation, including bread, but the Mediterranean diet doesn't shy away from eating carbs.

Vegetables are a hugely important when it comes to Mediterranean diets. It's not a vegan or vegetarian diet, but there is an emphasis on eating fresh produce that is grown locally. It's not uncommon to see locals gathering baskets of fresh vegetables or herbs, foraged in the local hills and countryside.

Legumes and grains are also encouraged in the Mediterranean diet. Some diets rely on cutting out high-protein beans, so some people find it rather surprising that these are allowed and even encouraged on the Mediterranean diet. With these included in the diet, perhaps you can begin to see why you'll never go hungry on this diet!

The Mediterranean diet aims to cut down on how much meat, especially red meat, you eat. There's an emphasis on eating fresh fish, although fish won't be eaten every day. As you follow the Mediterranean diet, you're encouraged to consume fish around twice a week.

Fruit is of crucial importance, when it comes to establishing a healthy Mediterranean diet. Whilst many diets try to cut out fruits, because they're high in sugars, those on the Mediterranean diet don't mind how much sugar might be in their fruit, as long as there's no added sugar.

The Mediterranean diet does allow some dairy consumption, though it is much lower than in other countries, such as the USA.

Eggs can be consumed, but usually just a couple a week, and mostly the whites when cooking with the egg.

Dairy, especially fats derived from dairy, like butter, don't feature much in a Mediterranean diet. Instead, the focus will go towards olive oil, as being the principal fat you cook with and drizzle over your salads.

Greek

A Greek diet is one that's most commonly thought of when someone starts discussing a Mediterranean diet.

It's clear that the Greeks have a good understanding of what to eat to maintain a healthy lifestyle.

Why do you think they're so often associated with beautiful gods and goddesses all the time?

Greek-inspired cuisine has made its way across the world, with many popular items such as moussaka appearing on numerous menus, despite what the type of cuisine at a restaurant might be.

Some people believe that the diets of those that live in Greece might be the healthiest in the world. This is country that has some of the lowest heart disease, Alzheimer's, and depression rates in the world. They're certainly doing something right.

Living on a gorgeous sunny island with an endless amount of beautiful sights probably helps, but a diet is important in maintaining a long and healthy lifestyle as well. Of course, the Greeks have a wonderful sense of community and place a high value on the importance of family too.

One common reason those in Greece have such healthy lifestyles is because of a surprising fact. They consume far more fruit and vegetables than the typical American.

The World Health Organisation (WHO) recommends eating at least 400g per day of fruits and vegetables. Greece has an average supply of 756 g per day of fruit and vegetables. By comparison, in 2015, just 9 percent of American adults met the intake recommendations for vegetables.

Before you start worrying about the idea of increasing the amount of vegetables you eat - it's easy, when you use a little Mediterranean know-how. Imagine a quiche, filled with fresh vegetables, a freshly baked zucchini or simple capers salad, with flavorful tomatoes, drizzled with olive oil.

There's an emphasis on cooking vegetables in olive oil or baking them with various herbs, so that the flavors simply burst on your palate with every mouthful.

Unlike many American homes, where take-out food, or convenience food is often eaten, Greek food is prepared fresh each day for the family.

Simple lifestyle choices like these have helped lead Greece as one of the healthiest countries on the planet.

In Greece, there is also a great emphasis on drinking water. Fresh bread and water is served with every meal, and a glass is always provided, even if someone doesn't ask for one in the first place. Drinking adequate amounts of water is vital for maintaining our health.

Lemon is another factor in what Greeks eat that make them so healthy. Lemon is an acid that can help aid in digestion, when added to any meal or even a glass of water.

Those in Greek culture only eat desserts occasionally. Sweets and other treats are saved usually for holidays or special occasions. Instead of eating too many sugary sweets, Greeks will kill their cravings with fresh fruits, such as grapes or berries.

Cyprus

Cypriot cuisine still has its roots in the Mediterranean diet, but there are a few different aspects that separate this particular country's cuisine from others.

There is more of an emphasis on meat dishes in Cyprus, versus other countries that tend to stay a little more traditionally vegetarian. Meat is usually prepared in slices and often grilled. The way that it is cut and cooked serves a purpose.

Traditionally, families would have to make their meat stretch across a longer period of time. Instead of cutting meat into chunks, it was cut into slices in an attempt to make it last just a little longer.

From this tradition has sprouted the idea of many kebobs, and other meats on sticks that are often cooked over an open flame.

The food around the island of Cyprus includes plentiful amounts of rice and pasta, beans and lentils, and fresh Mediterranean vegetables.

Turkey

Turkish cuisine is another one that is popular all over the world. The food in Turkey has similarities to that of Greece and Cyprus, though the flavorings involved differ.

Greek food will often be accompanied by a yogurt sauce, whereas some other traditional countries try to avoid dairy altogether.

Turkey is also known for providing delicious meat kebobs as well. Lamb is the most commonly consumed meat, though it isn't eaten as often as outsiders might believe.

Mediterranean Food Pyramid

Many of us were taught about the food pyramid when we were children.

The traditional food pyramid started at the bottom with grains, with less of an emphasis on other food groups until the very small portion of sugar was met at the top.

For years, this has been taught to generations of Americans as what they should be eating. However, in recent years, doubts have been raised about just how 'healthy' the food pyramid really is.

The Mediterranean diet has its own pyramid that many believe is a better example of what a healthy diet should include.

What differs in this model is that not every section is what a person should be eating either. Instead, there is an emphasis on physical activity.

This particular pyramid was made in 1993 as a healthier alternative to the U.S. pyramid that already existed.

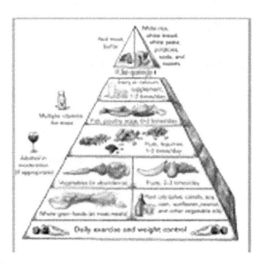

The pyramid starts at the bottom with an emphasis on physical activity and connection socially with other people. This includes dancing, laughing, or just simply expressing feelings with other people.

There aren't many other food pyramids that include physical activity such as this, but it's a crucial part of maintaining a healthy diet and lifestyle.

The next step up is the core foods that should be eaten each day. These include foods, such as vegetables, whole grains, fruits, and healthy fats, such as olive oil. These foods are all equally important.

After the core foods are listed, the next step up is fish and seafood. These are healthy foods, but they should only be eaten two or three times a week, not every day like the foods below them.

The same goes for any foods that include dairy. These foods are OK to eat on a Mediterranean diet, but shouldn't be consumed every single day.

Red meat and sweet foods are at the very top of the pyramid. These are foods that are not often consumed on a Mediterranean diet. They don't have to be eliminated, but they should only be eaten rarely, perhaps once or twice a month.

Red meat should be treated like sweets, only consumed from time to time. It doesn't have to be completely limited from someone's diet, but should be avoided as much as possible.

At it's most simple, the Mediterranean pyramid helps you focus on how often certain foods should be eaten, rather than what portion of each you should be consuming.

2

WHY THE MEDITERRANEAN DIET?

When choosing a the diet for you, you've probably been faced with an endless amount of options.

You could go for the diet that the person on your social media account is telling you to try. Maybe they make others perceive that they have a perfect and flawless life, so they'll convince you to start on their diet.

All you have to do is use their discount code to order the supplements online! Once they finally get to you, you might realize that these can cause heart conditions and may have a very low chance of actually helping someone lose weight.

This diet might not work, so you decide to finally try the one that your mother has been calling you about. Hers involves making gallons of cabbage noodle soup, which will act as a cleanse.

You might try this for a couple of days, but soon you'll find that you're hungry all the time and spending too much time on the toilet. That's two diets that still haven't worked, but hope is not lost yet.

Maybe you go to the store and see some new supplements in the health section. This diet is different though. It's not about taking a pill, but instead drinking something before every meal you eat!

It works, as long as you drink it directly before eating and are okay with almost gagging up the liquid every time you have to chug a bottle. Oh, and did I mention you only get to eat once a day on this diet?

There are so many diets someone can try when they want to change their lifestyle. The unfortunate part is that most of these techniques and tactics won't stick.

The reason is that they're just way too hard. They offer little interest and even less nutritional value, causing little payoff after very hard and strenuous work.

The Mediterranean diet doesn't involve any of this pain or stress. The answer isn't found online in expensive supplements, and you sure won't find it in your mother's diet books.

Best of all, you can buy what you need for this diet at any store, right in your very own produce section.

More Than a Fad

Many diets come and go, but the Mediterranean diet is here to stay. In the 1960s, scientists discovered that the people in Mediterranean countries were much healthier than anywhere else in the world.

Since then, the foods that they eat and the things that they do throughout their day became inspiration for many areas of nutritional study. Those that have tried living by the Mediterranean diet usually find their overall health improving in ways they never thought possible.

What makes this diet more than just a fad is that when you start sticking to this diet, you'll have trouble going back to the way things used to be. Your body will become accustomed to eating healthfully and you'll feel the impact of making poor diet choices or eating sugary foods.

The reasons why so many other diets come and go is because no one actually enjoys being on them! After just a short time on the Mediterranean diet, it won't feel like you're on a diet at all. You'll start to eat healthier and full of vitality. You'll probably find that you're beginning to enjoy life more too!

When you start on the Mediterranean diet, it won't be long until you fall in love. The foods you'll start enjoying might be new to you at first, but they're so full of flavor and goodness, that you'll soon learn to love them, as much as the Italian, Cretans and French do.

Of course, the Mediterranean diet is more than just a way of eating. It is a lifestyle. It's a good habit that, once established, can be hard to break away from.

People stick to the Mediterranean diet because it not only works, but they have a good time while dieting. Best of all, it doesn't really feel like a diet at all, it just feels like eating good, fresh food that tastes great.

Backed by Research

The Mediterranean diet isn't just the latest fad diet, or something that's being shared on social media. It's not a diet thought up by a random person to sell a product and make money off their book or ideas.

The Mediterranean diet is a way of life that people have been living for hundreds of years.

Once scientists discovered how healthy the people that followed a Mediterranean diet were, they took it into their own hands to start discovering what it was that made this idea so healthy.

There is research being done on the Mediterranean diet, with one source stating that the Mediterranean diet[1]:

"has been reported to be protective against the occurrence of several diseases. Increasing evidence suggests that the Mediterranean could counter diseases associated with chronic inflammation, including metabolic syndrome, atherosclerosis, cancer, diabetes, obesity, pulmonary diseases, and cognition disorders ....

The Mediterranean diet has been considered for the prevention of cardiovascular and other chronic degenerative diseases focusing on the impact of a holistic dietary approach rather than on single nutrients.[2]"

Tested by Millions in Mediterranean Countries

While certain isolated studies help to showcase the advantages of the Mediterranean diet, there are millions that live in the Mediterranean that are proof that this diet works best.

They live longer lives, are more fulfilled fulfilling experiences and have a great quality of life.

People in Mediterranean countries have a lower risk of experiencing heart disease or inflammation.

That is because a Mediterranean diet puts emphasis on anti-inflammatory foods, reducing inflammation in many people that choose to switch to this diet.

Those who follow a Mediterranean diet also have a lower report of chronic pain and illness. This might be because of the inflammatory properties, but it can also be linked to the idea that whole foods provide the body with more nutrients needed for smooth bodily functions.

Reports of uterine cancer are also reported to be lower in Mediterranean countries.

The chance of developing breast cancer is 68 percent less in Mediterranean countries, with women in the Mediterranean reporting fewer cases of breast cancer.

Those are some pretty impressive statistics that are enough for many people attempt a Mediterranean diet.

Brain power is overall boosted when a person chooses to partake in a Mediterranean diet. They no longer have brain fog that comes along with processed foods that can disrupt memory and other functions in the brain.

Super-fruits and hearty vegetables can increase brain function and decrease inflammation in other areas of the body. When brain power is boosted, this also helps in the aging process. This is likely why there are less reported instances of Alzheimer's disease.

Not only do people age more slowly mentally, but they physically last longer as well. A healthy diet and exercise are emphasized as a natural part of life, not just something that you should do if you have the time.

There's a real emphasis on relaxing or eating outside with family members. At homes and restaurants around the Mediterranean, the emphasis is on eating together with friends or family, laughing and sharing stories together. It's a far cry from having a quick burger from your local drive through.

Exercise doesn't mean paying out big for a gym card either. Life around the Mediterranean makes it easy to incorporate exercise into the daily routine - from walking to the store, meeting up for a coffee with a friend, pulling weeds in the garden, or simply going for walks in the surrounding countryside to gather fresh herbs.

No Deprivation and Reduced Cravings

If you've struggled with feeling deprived on other diets, this is the diet for you. You don't have to give up eating, starve yourself or sacrifice tasty foods for tasteless soups or smoothies. You're encouraged to eat until you're full, so that you don't' overeat or snack too much throughout the day.

There are so many delicious foods that you can eat while on a Mediterranean diet, that you won't feel like you're really having to give up too much.

You can still eat bread, cheeses, and certain meats. You may find it challenging to give up sweets, but once you get past the first week, you'll find those cravings will almost vanish.

Mediterranean diets encourage people to sit around a table and share stories with friends while eating. Why not try to encourage friends and family to join in with your new 'diet'?

There is an emphasis on family gatherings on a Mediterranean diet, so it's a great path for some families and groups of friends that are all looking to diet together.

The Mediterranean diet helps with the overall reduction of cravings. You're encouraged to eat throughout the day, rather than focus on one huge meal right before bed.

Snacking on nuts and fruit is encouraged. Having four or five small meals is preferable to eating two massive ones and maybe a small one.

Meals shouldn't be skipped, as they shouldn't just be seen as time to eat. Think about each meal as a chance to connect with those around you, or simply as a time to contemplate life.

On the Mediterranean diet you won't have to:

- count your calories

- eat tasteless food you don't enjoy

- weight out your foods

- starve yourself

As long as you don't continually stuff yourself and continue to make smart decisions, a Mediterranean diet will work.

Denying your body the very things that it is asking for is not going to help anyone in the long run. The Mediterranean diet encourages you to eat as much as you want, as long as you're not doing so in an unhealthy way.

Works with your Hormones

One of the greatest parts about a Mediterranean diet is that it works with the body. It doesn't force the body to do anything it shouldn't do, like go into starvation mode.

In fact, it's almost as if this is the diet that our bodies are supposed to live by.

The Final Diet

The Mediterranean diet is likely to be the final diet that you ever try.

If you commit to this diet, you'll realize that all the other things you've tried in the past were a waste of time.

This diet allows you to live the life you want without compromising too many of the things you want. It's a healthy lifestyle that's more than just a diet to help you lose weight.

Not only will you be happier and healthier, but you can also prevent other parts of your body from serious harm as well.

Let's take a look at the science behind the Mediterranean diet and the health benefits you might expect, when you follow it.

1

  https://www.researchgate.net/publication/261956692_Health_Benefits_of_the_Mediterranean_Diet_An_Update_of_
  Research_Over_the_Last_5_Years

2 https://www.ncbi.nlm.nih.gov/pubmed/24778424

3

THE SCIENCE BEHIND THE MEDITERRANEAN DIET

It's clear from various studies and actual experience that a Mediterranean diet has many significant health benefits.

This diet, which includes generous amounts of plant-based foods, offers many reasons why a person might choose to live a Mediterranean lifestyle.

In this chapter, we're going to discuss the health benefits that scientists have discovered about the Mediterranean diet.

As we go through these statistics, please remember that this is still about chance. We've all heard of the person who smokes and never exercises, who lives to be 100 years old.

Statistics are just that, statistics. Statistics are about chance and likelihood. There's no guarantees, just a higher chance of getting the benefits and outcomes you desire.

That said, let's start by taking a look at just one of the scientific studies:

"The Lyon Diet Heart Trial in 1998 showed that after three years on the Mediterranean diet subjects had a 56% lower risk of dying and a 50% to 70% reduced risk of myocardial infarction.[1]"

That's a 50% decrease in the likelihood of a death or heart problems, that's an astonishing statistic. If they had a drug that made that kind of impact, you'd be at the door clamoring for your physician to prescribe it for you.

In a society where we live longer, it's more important than ever that we retain our mobility and cognitive function. On the Mediterranean diet, overall function and mobility are increased, as well as the ability to age more slowly, compared to other cultures.

One of the reasons a Mediterranean diet is so helpful for so many different conditions is because of its anti-inflammatory properties. Inflammation impacts many of today's diseases, not least of these is arthritis.

Arthritis

Arthritis occurs when there is a painful inflammation and stiffness in the joints.

Some people associate arthritis with a lifestyle. They might believe that what a person does for a living is an indication of what their joints might end up like as they get older. That can be true.

However, there have been recent studies conducted that suggest what a person eats can significantly reduce the side-effects of arthritis.

Arthritis can be incredibly painful because patients can't bend or use their joints. It can be a debilitating disease and even the strongest pain medications can't always make it go away.

When it comes to living a Mediterranean diet, there is hope for anyone living with arthritis.

On the Mediterranean diet, you'll be eating more of the foods that will directly decrease inflammation and cutting out some of the foods which can cause inflammation.

A study was conducted that proved that some patients that stuck to a Mediterranean diet were able to significantly improve their physical function and feelings of vitality[2].

Patients that had arthritis and started a Mediterranean diet found that they no longer had joint swelling or inflammation. The foods that they were eating helped lead to their recovery.

It seems incredible that just changing up one's diet can reduce chronic pain so significantly.

No one should have to feel pain, by doing simple tasks that require the use of their hands. It seems that the Mediterranean diet might help anyone that struggles with arthritis and joint pain.

Incorporating part of a Mediterranean lifestyle can significantly reduce inflammation. It's all about choosing the right foods.

Whole foods, organic produce, and foods that are rich in antioxidants will help in reducing inflammation, but only when they are substitutes for the junk food and fatty food that you might have been eating before.

It's not just about using these healthy foods as a medicine, but using them to replace the foods that you already eat, the foods that you already know aren't so healthy.

It can be hard for anyone struggling with a painful condition to try something new. Who has the time to start a new diet? When you're struggling with chronic pain, it can be hard to make the change.

Anyone with arthritis may find significant relief from the pain in their joints. Although it might be hard to start a new diet in the beginning, in the end, it could be well worth it.

Asthma

About one in 12 people in the USA has asthma, that's about 25 million people. Between 2001 and 2011, the incidence of asthma increased by 28%[3]. That's a significant rise, with not much known about the cause of this increase.

Allergies include any form of coughing or wheezing, and for some kids, it can be as extreme as asthma and the struggles with breathing that involves.

A study of children in Crete noted that only a small percentage were affected by allergies. Researchers noted that the children in Crete with a low allergy and asthma rate also had a high access to organic fruits and vegetables[4].

A study was then conducted to determine if there was a correlation between healthy eating and healthy breathing.

What researchers found was that there was a distinct connection between low asthma rates and children that were put on more natural diets, such as the Mediterranean diet.

What's so great about this Mediterranean diet is that children will actually enjoy eating it. In fact, they may not even realise they're on a special diet at all.

They might still miss the candy and sugary sodas that they've become used to drinking, but the Mediterranean diet offers plenty of beneficial and tasty foods and drinks for kids to enjoy.

It might seem a little weird to put a child on a diet, but when it's a diet like a Mediterranean one, there's nothing to worry about, since it's not really a 'diet' at all. It's just a new way of eating.

Your child can still get all the proper nutrition they need without having to sacrifice too much. If eating more fruits and vegetables means having a freer airway and a healthier body, there's plenty of ways to encourage your child to sit down and finish their plate of greens or enjoy a smoothie.

No child should have to live with a condition like asthma. Luckily, the Mediterranean diet is there to help get them through.

Blood Pressure

A high blood pressure can be uncomfortable for anyone that experiences it. It can cause severe headaches or fatigue, cause difficulty breathing and, in extreme cases, stroke or even death.

What we know about high blood pressure is that it can often be reduced through diet and exercise.

It appears one of the greatest ways to reduce blood pressure is a diet that is consistent with the Mediterranean diet.

The Mediterranean diet reduces inflammation, stops insulin levels spiking, and promotes better digestion.

All those fruit and vegetables are packed full of micro-nutrients which work together to heal and repair your body and reduce inflammation throughout your body.

One of the reasons that blood pressure can be reduced is because of a high use of olive oil[5]. When you hear the word oil, you might start to worry, thinking that there is too much fatty acids in oil for it to be healthy. In reality, olive oil is a great fat substitute and has been directly linked to lower blood pressure.

On the Mediterranean diet you'll reduce your consumption of red meat, which can cause your blood pressure to increase.

Avoiding the triggers of high blood pressure is an important part of a Mediterranean diet, even for healthy patients that don't have blood pressure issues.

Unlike arthritis, high blood pressure doesn't cause continual pain, in fact, but it can still be very challenging to live with. Having to watch what you eat is never fun but on a Mediterranean diet, it's much easier, since it become a way of life.

The Mediterranean diet can be one of the tools used to manage your blood pressure, in discussion with your physician, of course.

You can enjoy eating nutritious food that actually tastes great. It's a way to reduce your blood pressure without having to subject yourself to the health risks of crash dieting.

Blood Sugar

Blood sugar is a measurement of how much glucose is present in the blood of a person.

For the typical American, your blood sugar levels are on a rollercoaster. Plummeting before a meal, then surging upwards with meals that are filled with sugar and fat, before coming crashing down again.

This isn't good, since when our blood sugar is too low, we can experience feelings of weakness, anger, hunger, and overall lethargy.

The rollercoaster of blood sugar levels can cause poor mood and can be a contributing factor to weight gain.

There have been studies conducted that show a direct correlation between a well-managed blood sugar level and a Mediterranean diet[6].

What's enlightening about this study is you don't need to count calories in order to manage your blood sugar levels. The only thing that's required to maintain healthy sugar levels is the Mediterranean diet.

At this point, you're probably starting to see just how much a Mediterranean diet can positively affect you and your body.

Once you feel the benefits, why would you choose to go back to stuffing yourself with sugar and feeling that high blood sugar haze?

Brain Health and Alzheimer's

Nearly 6 million Americans are living with Alzheimer's. Between 1999 and 2014, death rates from Alzheimer's climbed an astonishing 55%. Alzheimer's is one of the top 10 causes of death in the USA today.

When New York Citizens were studied for Alzheimer's compared to citizens in a Mediterranean country, the risk and diagnosed cases of Alzheimer's were noticeably higher in New York.

The biggest factor that differentiated the two groups of people, besides their geographical location, was the food that they ate on a daily basis. [7]

Those in New York were likely to eat fast food more often, or quick meals which were full of processed foods.

Those that were studied in Mediterranean areas focused their diets around fresh and whole foods. Processed meats, sugar, and dairy just didn't feature in their diet.

Another important factor in looking at what might cause Alzheimer's is the lifestyle of an individual, not just the food that they're eating.

Mediterranean cultures put a big emphasis on family time. Meals are more of a social interaction, rather than just eating quickly and getting done with your meal.

Interacting with others is important in developing and maintaining cognitive function.

Memory is often the first thing to go for people that find they have lowered brain functions.

Those that live a Mediterranean lifestyles choose to change things up, they eat smaller meals throughout the day, and enjoy having conversations with friends and family over their meals.

They enjoy and living in the moment, choosing to live life now, rather than focus on past regrets or anxieties about the future.

Cancer Fighting

In 2018, nearly 2 million new cancer cases were diagnosed in the United States, with over half a million cancer deaths[8].

It's all too common to hear news about a friend or loved ones diagnosis of cancer.

One of the challenges with cancer is that there is no exact way of determining what causes it, and, as yet, we're unable to completely cure cancer.

A Mediterranean diet has been associated with the reduction of the risk of cancer[9]. It seems that one thing that we can do is taking preventative measures, to reduce the risk of getting cancer in the first place.

Once cancer is diagnosed, a healthy diet may help to reduce the side effects, giving your body the nutrients it needs to repair itself.

Those in Mediterranean cultures are less likely to suffer from cancer, and if they are diagnosed, it is less frequently than those in other cultures, where the diets includes eating more fast foods and processed foods.

Processed foods are often linked to those that either have cancer or have a higher risk of contracting cancer. While not all processed foods will necessarily cause cancer, some processed meats have been classified as carcinogens.

Foods like hot dogs and lunch meats make up a huge part of the American diets. Few people seem to be aware that eating these foods might be putting them on the road to a cancer diagnosis further down the road.

One way to reduce the likelihood of this is to follow a diet based around whole and fresh foods, which is what the Mediterranean diet is focused around.

Cholesterol

High cholesterol can cause serious issues for many people. It can be an indicator that you're more prone to a heart attack or other serious health conditions.

While not everyone that eats unhealthily will get high cholesterol, it's certainly something to watch out for.

If you choose to follow a Mediterranean diet, you'll find it easier to reduce your cholesterol levels naturally.

This is because the diet is based less around foods that can cause high cholesterol, such as dairy, meat, and other heavy dishes.

Of course, those living in Mediterranean countries may still have high cholesterol, but it is less common than in other countries.

Mono-saturated fats are a big part of a Mediterranean diet. This includes nuts and oils that vegetables might be cooked in.

An increase in these mono-saturated fats in a person's diet have been linked to lower cholesterol, which in turn can lead to a lower risk of cardiovascular disorders and diseases.

Another key in reducing the chance of heart issues is red wine. While large quantities of alcohol can severely damage a person's body, red wine in moderation has been shown to be beneficial to your health.

Who wouldn't be happy to hear that a glass of wine each day can actually be good for you!

Depression

Depression is an illness that affects many people. The root cause of depression is unknown. Even seemingly healthy people can still suffer from depression.

The worst part about depression is that there is no complete cure.

Studies show that those who eat a Mediterranean diet, instead of foods higher in saturated fats and more processed foods[10], can reduce their risk of depression.

Of course, it's not just about what a person eats, the Mediterranean lifestyle is an important factor too.

Let's take a look at the Roseto Effect. Research carried out in the 1950's studied dozens of families from one southern Italian community, who migrated to Pennsylvania.

Doctors were astonished to find that there was hardly any depression in the village of Roseto, attributing it to the close-knit communities and support structures around them[11].

It seems that our relationship with those around us, affects our health. This was a landmark study, which rocked the scientific world. Scientists often study inputs and outputs, cause and effect, but our relationships are far harder to quantify.

The close-knit communities and family structures of the Mediterranean, can have a preventative effect on depression. Spending quality time with our friends and family more often, is a key aspect of living a more Mediterranean lifestyle.

Those living around the Mediterranean tend to spend more time outside, in the open air. When we're able to increase the amount of sunlight we let into our life, as well as spending time in nature, we're likely to have good levels of vitamin D, the 'sunlight' vitamin.

Not everyone lives in a warm area where they can sit outside, or even eat meals in the sun. There are supplements that can increase a person's vitamin D, but the best way to get more of this is directly from the sun.

Vitamin D3 promotes the brain's serotonin levels, promoting a 'feel good' factor, which can help those suffering with SAD[12] or depression.

Those that live a Mediterranean lifestyle know that it's key that they spend as much time outside as possible, so when the sun does emerge on even the cloudiest of days, they will make sure to spend some time in its bright beams.

Diabetes

More than 100 million Americans are now living with diabetes or prediabetes. In 2015, over 9% of the population had diabetes[13].

There are many reasons why a person might be diabetic, but diet and lifestyle play a key role.

No matter what the cause of diabetes might be, it can be very tricky to manage and keep under control once diagnosed.

One of the greatest ways to reduce the symptoms of diabetes is by managing your diet. By controlling what you eat, you can improve your management of your diabetes.

A Mediterranean diet will help you jettison foods that are high in sugar, and you'll cut out foods like candy, sodas and other junk foods.

Following a Mediterranean diet can be a good step in the right direction to start managing your diabetes. Filling your plates high with fresh vegetables, can help you feel full, without the need to resort to filling yourself with sugary foods.

One study concluded that a Mediterranean Diet, without calorie restriction, was effective in the prevention of diabetes in subjects at high cardiovascular risk. Compared with the control group, the incidence of diabetes was reduced by 52%[14].

For adults who had trouble managing their diabetes, it was found that their symptoms were significantly reduced once they started a Mediterranean diet.

If you are diabetic or pre-diabetic, always consult your physician or health professional, before making significant diet changes.

A Mediterranean diet based around whole foods can really help to manage and reduce the symptoms of type 2 diabetes.

Heart Health

The heart is one of the most valuable organs in our body. While everyone has a heart, not everyone has a healthy heart.

There are many factors as to why someone's heart might not be in the best shape. They could have a history of heart disease in the family, or perhaps they had a condition as a child that has led to a weaker heart in adulthood.

The biggest factor why someone might end up with a lower heart health is because of diet and exercise.

While eating healthy foods seems obvious, it isn't always the complete answer to improving someone's heart. Reducing stress and controlling things that might cause tension can seriously decrease the chances of having poor heart health.

Heart health is significantly better for those that practice a Mediterranean lifestyle[15].

This improvement isn't only because of the healthy foods that they eat, but also because they live a less stressful life.

One way to improve heart health is to eat foods rich in anti-oxidants, poly-unsaturated fats, and whole foods, meaning deriving mostly from one ingredient.

Foods that are high in trans fats and unhealthy oils are likely going to increase the chance of someone having health conditions, even when eaten in moderation.

A Mediterranean diet allows for all these factors. Someone that eats a Mediterranean diet reduces the amount of fatty foods that they eat, focusing instead on only things that are going to make them healthier in the long run.

The key to a healthy heart too isn't to just avoid fats altogether.

There are plenty of healthy fats that can actually help someone, including olive oil and different types of nuts that anyone on a Mediterranean diet can load up on.

Lifespan

It was the Cretans ability to life a full life at ages of 90 and above that first intrigued scientists and got them studying their diet.

It's not surprising to learn then, that those that practice a Mediterranean lifestyle live longer, on average, than those that don't[16].

Everything about our diet and lifestyle is important in extending our lifespan. Staying active and eating well, can increase the years that you're enjoying an active life, rather than experiencing significant physical decline.

In Mediterranean countries, it's not unusual to see older men and women talking or selling at the local market, enjoying a coffee at the local cafe, or out in the vegetable patch picking fresh, ripe tomatoes.

Older people are taking an active part in life, they're not relegated to the sidelines. They're active, not immobile. They're engaged with what's going on in their community and playing an active part.

The Mediterranean diet has been linked to an increase in protection of a person's telomere.

A telomere is something that sits on the end of a person's chromosome, which is crucial in life longevity. When the ends of a person's chromosomes become frayed, it can lead to a shorter lifespan.

If you want to protect your telomeres and prolong your life, a Mediterranean diet might just help you do that[17].

Of course, there's more to it than just your telomeres. Your heart health, mood, cholesterol, and risk of cancer will all be direct indications of how long you might live.

To live well, until you're 80 or 90, means eating well, looking after your body, being part of a community and having regular, physical activity.

Mood Boost

Many diets aren't great for your mood, either because you're not receiving proper nutrition, or because you end up starving yourself, causing crankiness and moodiness.

A study looked at individuals who were on a Mediterranean diet for ten days. They found that a significant percentage of individuals reported having a better overall mood[18].

Whilst you might choose a diet because you want to lose weight, what you might have overlooked is how your diet contributes to your overall mood.

You could put yourself on a juice cleanse and end up losing ten pounds in a week, but does that mean you'll also be happy at the end of the week? Maybe, maybe not.

One of the best ways to not only maintain a physically healthy lifestyle, but a mentally healthy one as well, is to include foods that will end up boosting your mood.

Mood-boosting foods include leafy greens, foods high in probiotics, and those that contain omega-3s.

Your serotonin level has a huge image on the state of your mental health. If you're are prone to depression and anxiety, it's possible that you have lower serotonin levels than others.

Leafy greens, like arugula and spinach include high levels of magnesium, which is crucial in maintaining or increasing serotonin levels.

Foods that have high probiotics, such as pomegranates and berries, can also help digestion. Our gut health is important in improving our overall health as well. How we treat our stomach will reflect how we're treating our brain.

Salmon is a great food, because it is full of omega-3s, that can help boost your mood.

Another key factor in improving your mood is your lifestyle.

Bringing home fast food every night, sitting in front of the TV while they eat, and ignoring your friends and family, might be a big reason why you struggle with low mood.

As you begin to follow the Mediterranean diet, start making some simple changes. Explore how you can enjoy eating outside more, and put an emphasis on eating leisurely meals with family and friends.

If you're an introvert, you'll need to have some time alone, but we're social creatures, made to be in community.

Sharing a meal is the way that people have shared in community since the dawn of time. If you can find a way to spend time enjoying meals, a glass of wine, or just a handful of nuts, with their friends and family, you'll be boosting your mood naturally.

A great way to ensure that mealtime is being shared with others is to plan on making meals together.

Why not get together with your friends and take turns providing different dishes?   Or plan in more meals with family and friends?

Weight Loss

The first reason anyone looks at a diet, is probably because they want to lose weight.

That might be the first reason, but hopefully from what you've already seen here, it won't be the last reason you consider the Mediterranean diet.

Over the last few years, obesity has been increasing at a phenomenal rate. In the 1960's obesity was almost unheard of, now, it's the norm, with even our children struggling with obesity.

We live in a society where how we look is important. If we're too fat or too skinny, we may not get the recognition we deserve.

Perhaps you feel inadequate and struggle with having a positive body image.

Too many people are willing to risk their health, just so they can lose weight. They dream of fitting into a certain dress or jeans, or they want to look good in photos.

Don't be tempted to compromise your health, just because you want to lose weight.

While losing weight might be your goal, there are plenty of other health benefits that come with following a Mediterranean diet.

Weight loss is a major reason why someone might follow a Mediterranean diet, and there is research to back the legitimacy[19]. Many people have found that their weight started dropping, once they followed the Mediterranean diet.

The best part about following a Mediterranean diet for weight loss is that it's not as difficult to follow as most other diets.

Some diet make you cut out everything that tastes good, in order to only eat foods that will cause fat decrease. That doesn't have to happen on a Mediterranean diet. Fruits and vegetables are encouraged, you can cook with delicious olive oil, and even drink red wine.

The key to the Mediterranean diet is moderation. There's no calorie counting or feeling hungry or deprived.

You'll find some recipes that you love to cook over and over again, that you'll really enjoy.

It's a diet that focuses on delicious foods that help and heal your body, promoting long-term health and wellbeing.

1 https://www.todaysdietitian.com/newarchives/050113p28.shtml

2 https://ard.bmj.com/content/62/3/208.short

3 https://www.healthline.com/health-news/children-allergies-and-asthma-on-the-rise-110813

4 https://thorax.bmj.com/content/62/8/677

5 https://academic.oup.com/ajcn/article/80/4/1012/4690349

6 http://care.diabetesjournals.org/content/34/1/14.short

7 https://onlinelibrary.wiley.com/doi/abs/10.1002/ana.20854

8 https://www.cancer.org/research/cancer-facts-statistics/all-cancer-facts-figures/cancer-facts-figures-2018.html

9 https://www.cambridge.org/core/journals/public-health-nutrition/article/mediterranean-diet-and-cancer/9DB8C2CE26619CD917F857E577DB8D0A

10 https://onlinelibrary.wiley.com/doi/abs/10.1002/ana.23944

11 http://yocuzlawyers.com/2011/06/the-roseto-effect-the-valley-of-the-roses/

12 https://link.springer.com/article/10.1007/s002130050517

13 https://www.cdc.gov/media/releases/2017/p0718-diabetes-report.html

14 http://care.diabetesjournals.org/content/34/1/14.short

15 https://www.sciencedirect.com/science/article/pii/S0140673602114723

16 https://www.nejm.org/doi/full/10.1056/nejmoa025039

17 https://www.bmj.com/content/349/bmj.G6674.full

18 https://www.sciencedirect.com/science/article/pii/S0195666310006963

19 https://www.nejm.org/doi/full/10.1056/NEJMoa0708681

4

SECRETS OF THE MEDITERRANEAN LIFESTYLE

The Mediterranean diet has been proven over decades to be an effective diet for weight loss and a healthy lifestyle.

But what about the Mediterranean lifestyle? How can you incorporate that into your life, without moving lock, stock and barrel to the south of France, Greece or Italy?

After years of traveling to Italy, France and Greece, there are lifestyle tips that I've noticed that I believe are a vital part of why the Mediterraneans live as well as they do.

Some of these may be obvious, but others may be less so. I include them here, as you may choose to incorporate some of them into your own diet and lifestyle.

One of the weird things about most diets, is that they forget that you're a whole person, far more than the sum of each individual part.

The Mediterranean diet recognised that you're a whole person. It's not just one thing we change that will bring about the benefits, but making small changes to each area of our life, that can really add up and make a difference to how we feel.

As we incorporate one small diet or lifestyle change at a time,   that's when we'll start see the benefits in our life, both in our health and our wellbeing.

We've looked at the some of the science behind the diet. We've seen how eating and living differently can impact your health, from your blood pressure to blood sugar levels, from your heart health to arthritis, and from preventing diseases such as Alzheimer's and cancer.

Let's get on with how we start to make these crucial differences in our life, by taking a look at the types of foods you'll be enjoying on a Mediterranean diet.

It's good idea to start with a personal goal, to ask yourself why you want to go on a diet.

Why not take some time to sit down and figure out what your 'why' is. Why do you plan on dieting? Is it because you're going to lose weight? Maybe you just want to have better skin or hair. Perhaps you want to improve your odds of avoiding a disease that has affected someone close to you? Or do you simply want to improve your health and wellbeing?

Whatever your reason for choosing a Mediterranean diet, it's best if you formulate a plan as to how you're going to achieve your goal. Of course, it all starts with the food that you choose to eat.

We're going to take you through the foods that are best to incorporate as part of your Mediterranean diet. We will also be discussing which foods to cut down or avoid, but don't let them worry you, there's still plenty of delicious foods you can fill your plate with!

In the next chapter, we'll take a look at what foods you might want to stock up on and buy in for your store cupboard or pantry.

For now, let's look at what types of food you'll be eating on the Mediterranean diet and why each of these foods is important.

Let me start by saying that none of this is rocket science. In fact, much of what follows may seem to you like common sense.

As we go through the list below, there may be things which seem obvious to you. However, there are likely to be one or two things which you didn't know which are the reason you're reading this book.

We've also incorporated action points at the end of each section, with ideas and suggestions as to how you can start making a difference today or in the next week.

OK, it's time to take a look some of the secrets of the Mediterranean diet.

Enjoy Fresh Food

If you walk into any village around the Mediterranean, you'll notice that the savvy locals prefer to buy their food from local markets.

They rise early to shop at the market, buying fresh fruits, vegetables and herbs that were picked at dawn that same morning. They buy bread, cheeses and meats from the same stalls every week. They know where their food was grown and often, they also know the person who grew it.

Most of all, when they buy from the local market, they know that the food is as fresh as it would be if they'd grown it themselves. Fresh food is definitely preferable to anything foods that are processed or packaged.

The main reason that food is processed is so that it will last longer. However, during that processing much of the goodness is lost, not to mention the preservative chemicals that are usually added. When something has a long shelf life, it may be good for your wallet and your wealth, but it may not be so good for your health.

When any food is picked and packed, it starts to lose it's vital nutrients within hours. Even supposedly 'fresh' food in your local store, may have been picked days, or even weeks ago.

Buying fresh food allows you to get produce, while it is still bursting with vitamins, minerals and micro-nutrients. When it's freshly picked, it's full of flavour and still retains many of the nutrients your body needs.

In most other spheres of life, we understand the simple equation that what you put in affects what you get out. If you put in good quality, you're likely to get good quality back. It's a universal truth.

However, when it comes to our bodies, it seems that we overlook this. When we're pressed for time, we just snack on whatever's to hand, not caring about the ingredients on the packet.

We're busy, so we buy the cheapest food, rather than best.

All of this adds up and our bodies count the cost. When we put cheap, mass-produced foods into our body, why be surprised when our body rebels and shows signs of sluggishness, weight gain or chronic illness?

As with everything else in life, the rule of what goes in, is what comes out, applies to us and our bodies. The better quality the food is that we eat, the better the outcome.

How can you take action today?

Where can you buy fresh food?

Is there a farmer's market or local market near you?

Is there any junk food that you're   putting into your body, that you might need to cut out?

Spend More of your Income on food

What might surprise you to learn is that, around the Mediterranean, rural and city dwellers alike, spend far more on their groceries than those in other nations.

In the United States, a typical household spends just 6.5% of their income on food. In the UK, that figure is 8.7% and in Canada it's 9.6%.

However, France, Italy and Greece, which all border the Mediterranean sea, spend 13.6%, 14.2% and 16.5% respectively[1].

That's almost double what the average American spends on food!

It's not hard to imagine that if you spend more on good quality fresh foods, that your body might reflect this, with better energy levels and improved health.

If you want to see results, do you need to re-prioritise your budget? Doesn't it make more sense to spend food to maintain your health, rather than spending it on expensive health care, once you've lost your health?

Put simply, what price do you put on your health?

How can you take action today?

Can you review your budget, to allow you to spend more on the foods that you're putting into your body?

Choose Organic Food

Going back to the lifestyle of those around the Mediterranean, it's not unusual in many gardens or front yards to see a small vegetable patch, filled with a variety of herbs and vegetables that are picked fresh each day.

This get a power combination, of both freshly-picked and organic food.

But is the whole organic movement just a hype to get us to spend more on expensive food stuffs, or is there any basis for the move to organic foods?

Let's hear what the scientists have to say.

One study[2] concluded that organic foods provide greater levels of a number of important antioxidant phytochemicals (that is, anthocyanins, flavonoids, and carotenoids).

The study showed that organic varieties provide significantly greater levels of vitamin C, iron, magnesium, and phosphorus than non-organic varieties of the same foods.

As well as being higher in nutrients, the study showed that organic foods were also significantly lower in nitrates and pesticide residues.

What these studies can't tell you is how much better organic foods often taste. Organic foods are often grown slower, taking longer to reach maturity, so that the food itself reflects that, with a deeper, more vibrant flavor.

If you've ever eaten an organic chicken and a battery-farmed chicken side by side, you'll have experienced this yourself.

If you've ever eaten a freshly-pulled organic carrot, you'll know that it's miles away from the flavour of a carrot that you'll find in your local store.

How can you take action today?

You may not be able to replace all your food with the organic equivalent, but could you make a start?

Is there one food you're currently buying that you can replace with the organic equivalent?

Green Vegetables and Herbs

Green vegetables and herbs make up a significant part of the Mediterranean diet.

On windowsills and in small plots around the Mediterranean, herbs are grown and picked fresh, just as the food is being prepared. You can't get any fresher than that!

Vegetables can help keep the digestive system working while using up a small amount of energy to be processed. Greens are easy on the body and have many other positive effects, with their anti-inflammatory properties.

Leafy greens and other green vegetables can be incorporated into your diet in a variety ways. They can easily be added to an omelet for breakfast or tossed into a salad for lunch. Greens can be put on a sandwich or mixed in with a stir-fry. Or you can throw in a handful of leaves into a smoothie. There is an almost endless number of options!

Eating leafy greens can help the heart work better and can improve brain function as well. Herbs also play a pivotal role in the digestive process. Leafy greens play a huge preventative role, and are especially good for reducing your risk of Alzheimer's.

Herbs are able to add flavor to a dish that might otherwise be bland. Herbs can take the place of salt and other processed seasonings, replacing them with something that's actually doing your body good.

How can you take action today?

Is there one leafy green or herb that you could start incorporating into your diet?

Eat Plenty of Fruit

You may have heard that some diets warn against eating too much fruit, because of the sugar it contains. They can assume that because fruit has a high sugar intake it will lead to higher weight gain.

While all food should be eaten only in moderation, fruit has some beneficial qualities that make it a big part of a Mediterranean diet.

Fresh berries are a big part of a Mediterranean diet, as they are lower in sugar than other fruits and also produce great anti-inflammatory properties. Some have even linked high intake of fruits as a reason that certain health issues have disappeared.

If you can't get hold of fresh berries, remember that frozen berries from your store are also packed with goodness, so stock up your freezer with those, when fresh berries are out of season. For those who have to watch their budget, that frozen berries can often be cheaper than fresh, even when the fresh fruit is in season!

Tomatoes are another fruit (yes, they're a fruit, not a vegetable) that are plentiful in the Mediterranean diet. Tomatoes are a powerful anti-oxidant that can reduce inflammation, as well as the risk of other underlying health issues. Tomatoes can be eaten fresh, or add a deep, rich flavour when added to a cooked dish.

Fruits, like tomatoes and berries, can be part of a diet that work to prevent diseases. These fruits provide our bodies with anti-inflammatory qualities that can reduce inflammation in your body.

As with anything, eat fruit in moderation, don't go overboard. The byword of the Mediterranean diet, is moderation. One thing you'll see right across France, Italy and Greece, is moderation.

How can you take action today?

In what way can you incorporate more berries or tomatoes into your diet this week?

Cook with Seasonal Foods

Many of the rural societies around the Mediterranean are based around eating what is available seasonally.

In the Western world, we've got used to eating fruits and vegetables all year round. Yet, often they're flown half way around the world, just to end up on our plate!

Fruits and vegetables are best eaten when they are in season. That's when they're fresh, full of flavour and nutrients.

Of course, it's possible to buy fruits and vegetables when they're out of season, but consider how far they've travelled and how long ago they were picked, before you do so.

Seasonal fruits and vegetables tend to grow during times when our bodies need them. Starchier vegetables grow in the winter when we feel the need for a little more meat on our bones to get us through the cold season.

In the summertime, when it's hotter and we're more susceptible to dehydration, vegetables provide nutritious salads, without heating up our bodies.

Seasonal fruits and vegetables are often cheaper, or on discount, at the supermarket. So take some time to track fruits and vegetables that are in season.

One final thought, if the skin is edible, the skin is where the most nutritional value is held. If it's organic, eat that skin, and let it do you good!

How can you take action today?

Are there any foods you're consuming that have been flown half way around the world?

Can you replace them with some foods that are in season right now?

Reduce Meat Consumption

If you enjoy meat, don't panic - you can still eat meat on the Mediterranean diet. But remember the mantra of the Mediterranean diet, all things in moderation.

High meat consumption has been linked to more serious health issues, including cardiovascular conditions and some types of cancer.

Recent research has shown that some processed meats have even been classified as carcinogens. This means that red meats that have been processed might cause cancer in some consumers.

By comparison, those who reduce their meat consumption, can see benefits for their heart health, reducing the risk of cancer, Parkinsons and Alzheimer's disease[3].

Those in the Mediterranean are known for eating meat less frequently or in smaller quantities.

Whether it's red meat or poultry, those on Mediterranean diets have a lower intake, than the typical American diet.

This avoidance of meat isn't for moral reasons, rather, it's just the way their diet has evolved over the years.

Of course, it helps that there is plenty of fresh fish in the Mediterranean sea, so that it's easy to regularly enjoy fresh fish on the Mediterranean table.

How can you take action today?

Can you start by replacing meat with fish at one meal?

Could you start by having a meat-free Monday and then move on from there?

Could you cut down on portion sizes for the meat on your plate?

Consume Wine - in Moderation

When you drive practically anywhere in southern Europe, you'll see vineyards covering the fields and mountainsides.

Grapes grow easily and wine is available in abundance. If you visit a typical European supermarket, instead of rows and rows of beers to choose from, you'll see rows and rows of local wines proudly displayed.

What may surprise you to learn is that not all alcoholic drinks were created equal. Wine is pretty much the only one shown to be beneficial to your health, when consumed in moderation.

Studies have shown that drinking wine, in moderation, has positive health benefits, unlike drinking beer and spirits[4].

Red wine has been linked to having anti-inflammatory properties. Not only is wine good for the body, but it's good for the mind.

Having a glass of wine, either with dinner or afterwards while relaxing, can help ease the mind and alleviate stress.

How can you take action today?

What type of alcohol do you usually enjoy drinking?

Why not buy a bottle of red wine, and enjoy a glass of wine with your meals this week?

Reduce your Dairy Consumption

Europeans love their cheese and milk products, but only in moderation.

Walk up and down any store in the south of Europe, and one thing will probably strike you. It's hard to find the milk! When you do, it takes up probably a fraction of the shelf size of what you'd find in a typical British or American store.

That's because, in Europe, the practice of adults drinking large quantities of milk is just not something you'll see. Kids, yes, but adults, no.

Those who live around the Mediterranean eat dairy, but in smaller amounts[5].

When dairy is consumed, it's in whole foods like goat's milk and cheese, Greek yogurt, or feta cheese. There's no added sugar, no added ingredients, just great-tasting food that's a joy to eat.

Take a look at some of the dairy products in your local store - how much sugar does that yogurt contain? How much sugar is in that 'milk' drink you sometimes enjoy?

Instead of a sugar or sugar-substitute filled yogurt, why not replace it with Greek yogurt, and top with a few fresh berries or freshly sliced fruit pieces?

How can you take action today?

How could you begin to replace the milk in your diet?

Are you eating any sugary milk products that you could replace with products without sugar, or a non-dairy option?

What products are you consuming that contain 'hidden dairy' products?

Drink Enough Water

We're told all the time that we need to drink more water, but many of us find it hard to consume enough water.

Health authorities often recommend that your consumption of water is eight 8-ounce glasses. That's about 2 liters of water per day.

Perhaps you've seen those before and after photos, of someone when their body was not getting enough water, to the 'after' shot, when they'd been drinking plenty of water each day. The impact of drinking sufficient water on our skin and wellbeing is undeniable.

If you find it hard to drink enough water, consider adding a slice of lemon, or a sprig of fresh mint. If that doesn't work for you, try chilling your water, as some people find that makes it easier to drink in larger quantities.

Walk down any European supermarket and there's often one or two aisles devoted to bottled spring water. Those living around the Mediterranean drink huge amounts of spring water, in preference to drinking regular water.

Spring water comes from ancient underground springs and contains natural minerals, such as magnesium, calcium, potassium and sodium, which our bodies need. By comparison, tap water is usually filtered or treated with chemicals to destroy bacteria.

Whatever type of water you choose to drink, unless you're drinking the full 2 liters per day, it's probably more important to increase your consumption, than to worry about what type of water you're drinking.

How can you take action today?

How many glasses of water do you usually drink in a day?

How could you increase this by one glass a day, this week?

Embrace The Mediterranean Lifestyle

The true Mediterranean diet is far more than just what you eat. It's also about your lifestyle.

What's going on our plate and into our mouth is important, of course, but there's so much more to us, than just our health. A lifestyle is about finding joy and fulfillment in our lives. It's about how we're living life, 24 hours a day, 7 days a week.

If you want to make real changes in your life, eating healthy foods isn't enough. Without addressing the issue of stress in your life, you're only addressing part of the whole picture.

Stress pervades every area of our life, damaging our minds and bodies. Our lifestyle, that is how we live each day, our day-to day-activities, affects our physical and mental wellbeing.

Your lifestyle includes the people that you regularly interact with, the job you work at, and the things you enjoy doing.

Those that live around the Mediterranean seem to have learnt how to prioritize their needs in a happy and healthy manner. They love to spend time outside, while exploring their surroundings.

Around the Mediterranean, you'll find a people that know how to work hard, and they know how to play hard. They value family, love socializing and know how to relax and switch off.

The Mediterranean people love spending time outside, whether that's lazing by the beach in the summer, pottering around the garden, or enjoying ski-ing in the cold of winter.

The cafe culture which is pervading around the world, started in these European countries, with people enjoying a friendly coffee with their neighbors.

Visit any village or town in Greece, and you'll see people sitting outside, chatting, people watching and enjoying a coffee together.

You'll see the same in France, on the streets of Paris. Socializing outside with friends and family, is just a natural part of the lifestyle.

During the holidays, the roads across France are at a stand still. Why? Everyone is traveling home, to see their families. They spend their vacations eating, drinking and laughing together.

This all can seem miles away from how we live, far from the shores of the Mediterranean, but there are aspects of the lifestyle that we can incorporate into our own lives, to start seeing the benefit.

So, how can you take action today?

Consider what you most value in life? Is it family, friendships and loved ones?

Take a look at your diary or calendar. If someone took a look at your schedule, would they know what was most important to you? If not, what changes can you make, so that your life more accurately reflects your values?

Exercise with a Purpose

Walk along a typical country road in Greece, and you'll see men and women, from their teens to their 70's or 80's busy in the fields or gardens, caring for animals, or harvesting the crops.

In France, walk through any village, and you'll notice that many gardens have a small patch for growing food to eat. You'll spot people of all ages, working outside, getting their hands dirty, whether that's repairing a roof tile or putting up a fence.

Across the Mediterranean, people aren't afraid to get out and about. In fact, they relish living life outside.

They're happy to take time out for a relaxed cycle to the local shop. They enjoy a walk to the market, or into the countryside, searching for local herbs to add to their lunchtime salad.

Where possible, they walk, instead of taking the car, with the walk being an enjoyable experience, in and of itself. This is in sharp comparison to the typical American way of life, where just about anything, from returning library books to posting a letter, can be done from the comfort of your car.

In much of the so-called developed world, we've created hobbies to keep ourselves busy. Yet, whilst these hobbies might add to the quality of our life, they are often sedentary and don't encourage us to be physically active.

Exercise is important for everyone, not just those of us that want to lose or manage our weight. Exercise helps build muscle. Muscles burn calories. It's a simple equation, but one that works.

Of course, exercise also enables us to build our strength and maintain our mobility, as we age and grow older.

There are two types of exercise you'll notice in the people living around the Mediterranean.

There's the kind of work you do, where exercise is the by-product. For example, digging in the garden to get ready to plant tomatoes.

There's also exercise which you undertake, because it's part of a fun activity. For example, swimming in the sea, or ski-ing down a snow-covered mountain.

In our busy lives, it seems we've compartmentalized exercise. Exercise is what happens when we go to the gym. We put exercise in a box, and don't take time to consider how we can more easily incorporate it into our daily lives.

Here's some suggestions to get you started on incorporating simple exercise into your everyday life:

- walk up the stairs, rather than take the elevator

- walk to the shop, rather than take the car or subway

- try your hand at the DIY job yourself, rather than phone a contractor

- get off the bus or subway, one stop earlier and walk the rest of the way

- grow a few herbs in your own pot or patch of land, rather than buying hydroponically grown herbs in the store

Walking is probably the easiest place to start, to add exercise to your life. It's an opportunity to observe the world around you, and is completely free to enjoy.

Wherever you are, whether you walk regularly, or always take the car, you can probably increase the amount you walk, fairly easily.

You can easily monitor your exercise with a smartphone, just search for the apps, or use the one which comes with your phone. Establish a baseline for your current activity (for example, the average number of steps walked each day). Then, just work out how to increase your level of activity each week, until you're happy with it.

How can you take action today?

Have you put exercise in a box? Is there a journey you could walk this week, instead of taking the car, subway or bus?

Are there any outdoor activities which you enjoy, that you haven't spent time doing for a while, and could re-start?

Embrace Family, Community and Mealtimes

One important aspect of a Mediterranean lifestyle is actually sitting down to dinner with other people.

Whether that's friends, family, or neighbors at a restaurant, dinnertime is important in growing and developing deep, meaningful relationships.

There's something special about spending time with friends and family, preferably over a meal.

In society today, there's an emphasis on doing things quickly. Convenience is a key selling point for many products.

Sandwiches and other meals are marketed for being handheld, so we can eat quickly and on the go.

Our lives are about convenience. When it's time to eat, we just grab one of these convenient meals or snacks, eat it as fast as possible, throw away the packaging and move on with our life.

There is also an emphasis on drive-thrus, with more and more restaurants opening up a convenient way for us to quickly order and pick up food that we can finish eating in the car before we even get home.

With delivery services that we can use with our phone, we can type in anything we want, place an order, and have it delivered to us within just a few minutes.

How often do we prepare our meal, then sit in front of the TV, not focusing on anything else, but the TV show and just unconsciously shovelling the food into our mouth?

By contrast, the Mediterranean lifestyle puts an emphasis on taking time, sitting at the table, enjoying eating your meal, savoring the flavors and talking with other people around the table.

How do they do find time for this?

Around much of the Mediterranean, a 2 hour lunch break is standard. That gives office staff and shop owners time to pack up, go home, cook a meal, eat at their leisure and then return refreshed to work.

In outdoor cafes, you'll see labourers and office workers alike, sitting with their colleagues, laughing and joking over a shared meal.

What a far cry from the typical lunch at work, where we grab some food in just a few minutes, before returning to work, guilty for even having take a break.

We're built for community. We need connection with those around us. It's vital for our mental health and wellbeing.

We can wonder how we can connect meaningfully with others, yet, often all we really need to do is to sit and share some food with some friends.

In Mediterranean countries, meals are an event, where everyone is involved. In the evenings, the meals are more leisurely, typically taking two or more hours over a meal, of three or more courses.

Picture a long table in the sunshine, it's laid for 10 or 12 people, with glasses of water and wine sat on the table waiting for the family to come together.

As the mealtime approaches, the family gathers - children, the grandparents, the parents and the extended family, all sit around eating, chatting and laughing together.

Cooking food is a vital part of the process. This might involve sharing recipes with others and working as a group to prepare a meal. They can make sure that they have to do less work by taking turns on different nights to have the responsibility of preparing certain dishes.

People can bond in the kitchen while preparing the meal. Cleanup is much easier when everyone is involved as well.

Meals aren't mean to be just about shoving food in your face to stop your stomach from growling. That's OK and necessary from time to time, but if that's the way you're eating all the time, you're not doing your health any favors.

When was the last time you ate with family? Could you plan a date in your schedule in the next few weeks? Perhaps you could make it a regular thing? It might require more work at first, but in the long run, it will be worth it.

If you're unsure where to start, how about having one night each week where you cook something delicious, and eat it, without any distractions? No TV, no phone, just the food and whoever is with you, or your own company.

How can you take action today?

Who do you enjoy sharing a meal with?

When did you last eat a meal with family or friends? Can you put something in the diary this month or next?

Could you be more intentional about your lunch break, and take time to really enjoy eating and savor your food?

Get Out in the Sunshine

The sun plays a vital part in our lives, it is vital for plants to grow, it can lift our mood and warm our spirits. Without the sun, we simply could not survive.

Whilst too much exposure to the sun can be dangerous, so can too little exposure. Vitamin D is vital for our health, it helps to control and reduce inflammation in our bodies and it's exposure to the sun that enables our bodies to make it.

Whilst we need the vitamin D that the sun produces in our bodies, many of us find it hard to prioritize spending time outside.

Our lives are confined to our apartments, houses or offices, and we can live life indoors and rarely get out in the sun.

There are plenty of ways to get more sun without having to move to the Mediterranean.

Just letting in a little bit of sun every day, or getting out into the sun, can really help really lift your mood.

Walking is a great way to get some fresh air and some natural sunlight. Your body produces more vitamin D when the sun is highest in the sky.

It's only the exposed parts of your body that can react to the sun and help create vitamin D, so roll your sleeves up, or wear clothes that give you maximum sun exposure.

In some more northern states or countries, the sun doesn't get high enough during the winter months to help your body produce vitamin D at all.

So, how can you deal with this? Not all of us can up sticks and move to the Mediterranean, after all!

When the sun is not too hot or dangerous, perhaps you could take a lunchtime walk? Just 20-30 minutes in the sunshine on a summer's day, could really help boost your vitamin D levels.

If you're not fortunate enough to live in the sunshine states or the Mediterranean countries, to get sufficient vitamin D, you may need to be intentional about it. With so much of our lives lived indoors, you may need to think about how you can get outdoors in the sun and what activity you can enjoy whilst doing so.

Your body stores vitamin D, so if you spend an extended period of time in the sun, your body can store it and use it over several weeks.

This means that there really is a long term benefit to taking a break or a vacation in the sunshine, beyond the fun and relaxation of just getting away from it all!

It should go without staying, but please be sun-aware and don't risk burning your skin or staying in the sun too long.

Maybe you have no idea whether you're getting enough vitamin D? One solution would be to ask your doctor or physician to do a blood test. You can also do a test at home, post it off and get the results in days. There's also an app that allow you to monitor your exposure to vitamin D, which can help keep you safe by warning you when you've had *too much* time in the sun. At the time of writing, Dminder is the app that I've found easiest to use.

If you live somewhere that you don't get enough natural vitamin D or can't afford a vacation to the sun, one solution is to take vitamin D3 supplements. These are an easy way to boost your levels of vitamin D. However, please check with your physician or health practitioner, before taking any supplements.

It's important to get outside in order to meet new people, see new things, and most importantly, get some sunshine!

How can you take action today?

If you live somewhere that it's dark during much of the day in the winter, could you get a blood test to see if a D3 supplement could be beneficial to you?

How can you be intentional about getting more sunshine on your body, when the days are long and the weather is warm and sunny?

Practice Mindfulness

Mindfulness is the process of becoming more aware of your surroundings. It's about living in the moment, rather than constantly focusing on the past or the future.

Mindfulness is a tool to ground us and bring us back to the present.

In our fast-paced world, it's easy to get caught up in everything. It's only natural to be anxious about the future. We're anxious for our finances, our family, our environment and the politics of our country.

While we're worrying about the future, we're also worrying about the past. If only we didn't spend that money at the bar yesterday, we'd have it to pay that bill today. If only we had studied something else in college, we might have a better job now.

We can worry that maybe we should have given that one date an extra chance. We could have missed out on "the one," after all! Or perhaps we have regrets about those people we did date and feel we should have broken up with them sooner to avoid a messy breakup.

Our minds are so busy, preoccupied with anxieties about the future and worries about the past, that we can miss the very moment we're experiencing right now!

The goal of being mindful is to look at the things around you right now and enjoy the present.

Mindfulness starts by becoming aware of your surroundings. It's a simple technique that you can use at any time or any place, to promote calm and wellbeing.

When you put emphasis on what's going on in the present moment, you'll learn that you can let go of the anxieties filling your head.

Imagine living in a small Greek village. You start your day with a coffee and breakfast, sat outside in your garden, surrounded by nature. As you walk to work, you greet your neighbours and chat briefly about your day. At the end of your day, you meet up with a friend for an hour or two, going out on your fishing boat.

Or perhaps you live in a busy French city. You take a leisurely breakfast, as you don't start work until 10am. After a couple of hours of work, it's time for your two hour lunch break. You walk home, spend time cooking a meal, and share it with a loved one. Back to work and you greet your colleagues warmly. At the end of your day, you meet up with a colleague for a relaxing coffee, then take the subway home for a leisurely meal with your family.

Sounds idyllic? How easy would it be to live in the moment, if our lives were only different.

But that's the wrong way of looking at things. What if you turn it on it's head. How would our lives be different, if only we could learn to live in the moment?

Not long ago, I walked along a picturesque Greek fishing harbour. As I did so, I noticed a small family, obviously on vacation. They were sitting at a waterside cafe, which had views of the cobalt blue sea and the verdant hills beyond. By any measure, it was an idyllic spot. Yet, each member of the family was sitting looking at their phone, failing to appreciate or engage with the beauty all around them. That family could certainly have taken a lesson of the benefits of living in the moment!

People living in Mediterranean countries worry less about their life, because they're too busy appreciating or engaging with what's around them. It's just a different way of living, perhaps with different priorities.

The first step in becoming mindful, is to become more aware of each moment. To enjoy the walk, the journey, the food or the people that you're experiencing right now.

It's about noticing the enjoyable moments as we go through our busy day. It's a choice, it might not come easy at first, but it can be easily learned, with practice.

How can you take action today?

Can you think of a time when you could have focused on something enjoyable, but your mind was focused on something else?

When your mind is pre-occupied, can you find something that you can focus on or do, that takes you away from those unhelpful thoughts?

Perhaps next time you're out with friends or family, you could try not using your smartphone. Instead, focus on those around you and what they're saying.

Set Time for Rest and Relaxation

Too many of us worry about everyone else, so much so that we forget to focus on ourselves.

We can put our emphasis on working hard, progressing at our company, and looking forward to the day when we retire. We can make big plans for our future retirement, whilst failing to appreciate the value of living our life right now.

You might be successful, but would you say that you're happy? How stressed would you say you are, compared to those around you?

What many people don't realize is that stress can have serious negative health effects. It can damage your heart, wreck your immune system, and wreak havoc on your stomach.

Of course, there will always be things that cause us anxiety. While many people push stress to the back of their minds, those living in Mediterranean countries have the best of both worlds, they work hard, but they also play hard. They work as hard at their times of relaxation, as they do at their job.

So, how do you begin to incorporate more times where you can rest and refresh your mind and body?

Those that live in Mediterranean countries typically emphasize rest and relaxation. They don't feel so pressured to meet certain goals or expectations, instead focusing on themselves and their family.

Could you start incorporating at least an hour a week to just completely relax? Why not find something that you absolutely love to do?

Maybe it's finally taking a yoga class, or just going to see a movie. Whatever you choose, recognize these moments as your own. Turn off your phone if you have to.

Make sure that you're putting specific time in every week to ensure that you're getting the proper rest and relaxation that you deserve.

We all have trouble letting go, but those living around the Mediterranean know that it's important to let things go, not just for their stress, but their overall health as well.

How can you take action today?

In the last week, when have you stopped and just relaxed for an hour or more?

What do you love to do, that you find relaxing?

How can you incorporate more times of relaxation into your life?

Next Steps

OK, we've covered pretty much all the secrets of the Mediterranean diet and lifestyle.

So, what are your next steps?

You may want to jump right in and start today. Or you may want to start taking small steps, one at a time.

Whatever you choose, make a decision today, which it will be and consider what your next steps are and how you can take action today!

1 https://www.vox.com/2014/7/6/5874499/map-heres-how-much-every-country-spends-on-food

2

https://web.a.ebscohost.com/abstract?direct=true&profile=ehost&scope=site&authtype=crawler&jrnl=10895159&A
N=50734051&h=TANcVwajOlZXzJA9yJ7lVUEEi5K05uExhR%2b3K8eArJ2EvLrArR2iRf%2btc0qW%2fVMVydJ
44FVJ5rn1uaz7HkCX5w%3d%3d&crl=c&resultNs=AdminWebAuth&resultLocal=ErrCrlNotAuth&crlhashurl=logi
n.aspx%3fdirect%3dtrue%26profile%3dehost%26scope%3dsite%26authtype%3dcrawler%26jrnl%3d10895159%26
AN%3d50734051

3 https://www.bmj.com/content/337/bmj.a1344.long

4 https://onlinelibrary.wiley.com/doi/full/10.1111/j.1444-0903.2004.00583.x

5 https://academic.oup.com/ajcn/article-abstract/61/6/1321S/4651207

LISA SCOTT

5

MEDITERRANEAN FOODS

Let's take a look at what you'll need in your Mediterranean cupboard, as well as what your shopping list will include, when you embrace this new way of eating and living.

Mediterranean Store Cupboard

Fill your pantry, store cupboard with foods that easily can be incorporated into many different types of meals.

As with any diet, there will come a day when you'll just want something quick and easy to eat.

This is where most people fall off the diet wagon and start eating junk food.

Having a pantry, freezer or store cupboard filled with the right ingredients can help you stick to your Mediterranean diet.

There are plenty of foods that you can buy in bulk that will last several months. The larger your pantry is, the less food you have to buy week to week.

Building up your pantry might take a while, as you may not have the budget to purchase everything on the list in bulk right away.

Start a week at a time if you have to. Maybe one week you buy a large bag of almonds, and the next you purchase a huge bag of walnuts. Buying these things in bulk may not be cheap, but you'll find that they can end up lasting months at a time.

You may even find that the best price for bulk buys is through buying on the internet - even when you allow for postage. Take a look at the costs in your local store and compare with the internet prices.

Once you've filled your pantry, it's easy to maintain. Although it might cost more than your usual budget to set up your pantry, you'll probably spend less every week going grocery shopping.

As you find your favorite meals, make sure to buy in the dry and frozen ingredients for these, so that you can cook them, whenever you feel like it. This is a great way to deal with any cravings you might have, simply by being able to cook something you know you'll enjoy.

Let's take a look at the sorts of things to include in your store cupboard.

Whole Grains

Whole grains are one of the most important foods in a Mediterranean diet. These include foods that have three main parts: the bran, the germ, and the endosperm.

Many "grains," such as white bread or bagels, won't have all three of these, so avoid refined foods.

Wholegrain foods are high in selenium, B vitamins, dietary fiber, magnesium, phosphorus, manganese, and iron. Each of these vitamins and minerals is vital for creating a diet that's good for your mental and physical wellbeing.

The mistake many people make when creating their diets is to include refined grains. There's a big difference here, as refined grains aren't going to provide proper nutrition for your body.

Eating more whole grains instead of refined grains can reduce the risk of type 2 diabetes, cancer, and heart disease.

Important whole grains include:

- Rice
- Couscous
- Oats
- Buckwheat
- Whole-grain rye
- Millet
- Spelt
- Quinoa

All these foods can be purchased in bulk, and they'll usually last several months or even years.

Here's a quick tip - if you're buying a loaf of wholegrain bread, why not slice it up and pop it in your freezer? Then you take out as many slices as you need, whenever you need them.

Wholegrains are one of the foundational foods for living a healthy Mediterranean lifestyle.

Nuts and Seeds

Nuts are energy-dense foods. They're rich in bioactive compounds, macronutrients, micronutrients and phytochemicals.

If you're allergic to nuts, please just skip this section and move on to the next one.

Nuts are part of a heart-healthy diet. Nuts are full of 'good' unsaturated fats, that are thought to be beneficial for your cholesterol levels. They are packed with protein and minerals that are vital for our body to function well.

You might be used to eating processed nuts, with a high sugar or salt content. If so, you're adding a lot of extra salt and sugar to your diet, not to mention that you're missing out on the flavor and taste of nuts, picked fresh.

Here are some of the most important nuts to include in a Mediterranean diet, though there are plenty of others not listed:

- **Almonds** – Almonds have been directly linked to reducing cholesterol and are important in maintaining a healthy heart.

- **Hazelnuts** – these can be used in many sweets. While shop-bought chocolate spreads can contain nuts, they also contain sugars and fats that aren't so good for you. Why not try making homemade hazelnut spread instead?

- **Pine nuts** – these are great to include in different sauces, especially pesto. Pine nuts help suppress appetite and improve vision because of the high amount of cholecystokinin and lutein present.

- **Pistachios** – pistachios are another great nut that can be included in both sweet and savory dishes.

- **Walnuts** – these are great because many people that have peanut allergies won't be allergic to these. Walnuts are great to add to sweet dishes like cakes or pies, and savory dishes like pasta and salad.

- **Cashews** - these are rich in iron, zinc and magnesium, which has been linked to improved memory recall. Cashews are great to nibble on, when you're feeling a little hungry and need a snack.

Fresh Foods

Fresh is always better when it comes to picking out food from the store. Of course, fresh foods don't last as long, so you'll have to plan your menu carefully, so as not to waste them.

Take a look at the 14-day plan in Chapter 8, for some ideas of what and how to plan your meals.

Moving to the Mediterranean diet will mean that you'll probably be buying more fresh fruits and vegetables than you used to.

Personal preference is key here, but just because you're not sure if you like something doesn't mean you shouldn't still buy it.

You may not love spinach, but that doesn't mean you can't eat it. You could blend it into a smoothie or cook it in a large stir-fry, most of the time not realizing it is there once you start eating! Start with a few leaves at a time and then build up your tolerance to the taste.

You can make fruit and vegetables last longer, by storing them somewhere cool. You could even keep them in the fridge, if you have room.

To avoid waste, when you find that your fruit and vegetables are going bad too quickly, you might try using them in recipes to help elongate their life.

You could cut vegetables up and put them in chicken stock to make vegetable soup. This can be jarred and stored for later use. You could also pickle many different vegetables, and fermentation can seriously help digestion as well.

If your fruit seems like it's starting to turn bad, you can cut it up and cook it with just a little sugar and lemon juice to make a fruit spread. This could be enjoyed on toast, crackers, or as a topping on ice cream. Or you could just stew the fruit and serve with a drizzle of cream.

You could also take fruit that's ripe and blend it together with a little coconut milk. Freeze, and turn it into a delicious sorbet!

Food List

Let's take a look at how you can make following the Mediterranean diet easy for yourself.

First, we'll look at the food you should eat more of, which means that you should focus your most energy on this. If you eat only foods that are in that section, even better.

Then, we'll take a look at the foods that you'll need to cut back on.

Finally, we'll look at the foods that should be avoided altogether. These foods don't offer any health benefits, and most of them actually damage your body.

Eat More of These Foods

Below are foods that you can eat as much of as you want, remembering the rule, 'everything in moderation'. All these foods have specific benefits that will improve your overall health.

Here are foods that you can eat as much of as you like:

Vegetables

This includes:

- Artichokes
- Arugula
- Bell peppers
- Broccoli
- Cabbage
- Eggplant
- Garlic
- Green beans
- Mushrooms
- Olives
- Onions
- Peas
- Spinach
- Squash
- Tomatoes

Fruits

This includes:

- Apples
- Apricots
- Avocados
- Bananas
- Berries
- Cherries
- Dates
- Figs
- Grapes
- Lemons
- Melon
- Plums
- Pomegranates

Beans

This includes:

- Hummus (to make it yourself, please see the recipe included later in this book)
- Chickpeas
- Lentils
- Pinto beans

- White beans

- Garbanzo beans

- Black beans

Nuts and Seeds

- Almonds

- Cashews

- Flaxseed

- Peanuts

- Pine nuts

- Pumpkin seeds

- Sunflower seeds

- Walnuts

Oils and healthy fats

- Extra virgin olive oil

- Avocado oil

- Canola oil

- Grape seed oil

- Coconut oil

Fish and Seafood

- Clams

- Cod

- Crab
- Salmon
- Scallops
- Shrimp
- Tilapia
- Tilapia
- Tuna
- any fresh fish

Dairy and eggs

- Eggs
- Feta cheese
- Greek yogurt
- Low-fat and skim milk

Herbs and spices

Here's some of the typical herbs used around the shores of the Mediterranean:

- Basil
- Bay leaves
- Chiles
- Cilantro
- Coriander
- Cumin
- Mint

- Oregano
- Parsley
- Pepper
- Rosemary
- Sage
- Tarragon
- Thyme

Cut Back on These Foods

You might be used to eating some of these foods at almost every meal, but doing so could be damaging your health.

You won't have to completely eliminate these foods from your diet, but you should still to try to consume these no more than twice a week.

- *Poultry* – this meat is much healthier than other options. You can still consume food like chicken and turkey, but do so in moderation and buy organic, if you can.

- *Cheese* – cheeses such as feta cheese can help elevate a meal and add flavor, but this too should be consumed only in moderation.

- *Milk* - Any whole dairy, like whole milk or heavy cream, should be eliminated and replaced with almond or soy alternatives.

- *Red meat* – red meat is the hardest for the body to digest, so it should only be eaten infrequently. Some processed red meat has even been linked to the possibility of cancer

Avoid These Foods

The foods in the following section should be avoided, where possible. That shouldn't stop you from eating them, on the odd occasion, but if you're really looking to live a healthier lifestyle, these are the foods that you'll want to cut down or eliminate from your diet.

It can be a bit of a change to cut these out of your diet, so we've offered alternatives for you, so you don't have to feel as though you're giving up too much.

Beer and liquor– these can be hard for some people to give up. Many of us enjoy coming home and opening up a fresh beer. Eating a Mediterranean diet doesn't mean that you can't have a drink. You can still drink liquor every once in a while, but you should try to do so straight or on the rocks in order to avoid any added sugar that might be mixed in some cocktails. Red wine is a far better option. you can still drink white every once in a while, but red wine has been shown to have the greatest health benefit.

Salt – if you can, cut out table salt altogether. Table salt has been treated so that all the beneficial compounds are removed. Instead, replace with sea salt or a natural salt. Going Mediterranean doesn't mean that you have to give up on flavor. Instead of salt, try reducing the salt you add, and add in different herbs and spices to take a meal to the next level.

Butter – is undeniably delicious. Sadly, it's also not so very good for you or your health. Giving up butter doesn't mean giving up flavor, or any of the comfort foods that are found in butter. Healthy fats, such as olive and coconut oil, are still allowed in a Mediterranean diet, so choose these over butters. Any good cook knows that a small splash of butter can turn something from ordinary, to sublime, just don't do this everyday!

Chips – many people love chomping on chips when they're watching TV or doing something else that might require a snack. While most chips are processed with different saturated fats, that doesn't mean you have to give up on all chips. Instead of buying a bag at the store, instead try to make your own, such as kale or sweet potato chips. If you don't want to have to make your own, try eating more nuts as a snack instead.

Sugary or fruit drinks – These can be the hardest to give up. Many people love going to the local coffee shop and loading up on seasonal drinks. Unfortunately, these are often filled with unhealthy sugars that can cause health problems. Instead of drinking sugary coffee, try all-natural tea. Instead of soda, try drinking carbonated water. You can add fruit to both of these for flavor.

Cookies, candy, and sweets – This is the hardest thing to give up for most of us. Giving up candy and other sweets just means that you can't buy what's packaged at the store anymore.

Instead of eating a bag of your usual candy, try eating some roasted hazelnuts with a little bit of cane sugar and cinnamon. Instead of eating a package of twizzlers, try drying strawberries or making your own fruit leather. One easy solution is to carry with you some 'emergency' snacks, for when you need a sugar hit. Include nuts and dried fruits and carry with you at all times, for those snack emergencies!

Just a reminder here, you may be giving up some of your favorite foods, but you'll also be giving up some of the health problems that come with them!

OK, let's explore one of the diets that's hit the headlines recently. That's the Keto diet.

Just how easy is it to 'tweak' the diet to become a keto diet – how much of the Mediterranean diet fits well with a Keto diet?

LISA SCOTT

6

THE KETO MEDITERRANEAN DIET

The Keto diet is hugely popular. It's often seen as a quick way to lose weight.

If you're keen to lose weight quickly, here's some ideas to combine the Mediterranean diet with the keto method for quick results.

Ketosis is a state of digestion in which the body uses fat as an energy source. In everyone's body, the main energy source comes from carbohydrates. The body takes these carbohydrates and breaks them down into glucose, powering the body.

That's why, in an old version of a food pyramid, breads and grains are at the bottom. These are foods that are filled with carbohydrates the most. Foods like cereal, bread, and potatoes are loaded with carbohydrates that can provide a body with plenty of energy.

The problem with carbohydrates, however, is that they can be filled with sugar. Too many foods that are high in carbohydrates will result in a person gaining weight.

When the body has more carbs than it needs to provide the system with energy, then it will start to turn those carbohydrates into fat cells. This is why so many people might struggle with their weight; it is because their body keeps storing all the carbohydrates they eat.

The point of entering ketosis is that the body no longer stores carbohydrates as fat cells. Instead, the body uses fat as its primary energy source.

In order for this to happen, the body can't be provided with carbohydrates. When these carbohydrates are removed from the diet, the body looks for something else to get energy.

Then the body starts taking those fat cells and burning those down into ketones. The ketones then become the primary energy source, resulting in a massive amount of weight being lost.

Fasting has some health benefits, but can have just as many negative side effects. The point of fasting is to starve the body, and in a way a ketogenic diet does just that. Instead of having to starve, however, a person on a ketogenic diet can continue to eat as many fatty foods as they want.

A person on a ketogenic diet loads up on good fats, however, not bad ones. This provides the body with an energy source without having to add extra weight.

A ketogenic diet can include plentiful fruits and vegetables that are low in carbs. So, there are some similarities to the Mediterranean diet.

Although most vegetables will be OK on a keto diet, a lot of fruits are high in carbohydrates, so it's only the berries that you can include when on a Keto diet.

While a Mediterranean diet emphasizes whole grains, anyone on a keto diet cuts out grains altogether.

Here's some reasons why you might want consider a Mediterranean keto diet, at least for a short period:

- **To lose a massive amount of weight**. Anyone on a ketogenic diet will break down fat and use that as an energy source.

- **To prevent and treat cancer.** Both a Mediterranean and a ketogenic diet have been linked to helping prevent of some types of cancer. Please check with your physician, before changing your diet, especially if you have been diagnosed with cancer.

The main difference between a keto and a Mediterranean diet, aside from the intake of carbs, is that red meat is positively encouraged in a keto diet.

Is it really possible to combine the Mediterranean diet with the Keto diet?

Let's take a look at the high protein foods that you can eat on the Mediterranean diet. These include:

- **Seafood and fish** – this will provide the body with a healthy fat while still staying true to a Mediterranean diet that aims to reduce red meat. Salmon is probably one of the best foods that a person that wants to enter ketosis might want to choose.

- **Lean meats** - such as chicken or turkey

- **Low carb vegetables** – a Mediterranean diet encourages veggies of all kinds, but on a keto diet you have to be more careful about how many carbs you're eating. Low carb vegetables include broccoli, kale, and cauliflower.

- **Low carb fruits** - such as berries, but it's best to avoid starchy or sweet fruits, such as bananas or apples

- **Salads** - around the Mediterranean, salads are sublime. Get creative and go for fresh leaves, add in tomatoes, olives or feta cheese, for plenty of flavor.

- **Eggs** - these are so versatile, that you probably won't feel you're on a diet at all

- **Avocados** - in a class of their own, they're fatty and tasty, great to add flavor to any meal

- **Cheese** - include cheese like feta cheese, that add protein and can easily be added to a salad

- **Red wine** - the odd glass or two, will make the entire idea of dieting more palatable!

- **Fatty oils** – the healthier the fat, the better for a ketogenic diet. A Mediterranean diet will also focus on cutting out other fat sources, like butter, and instead focusing on oils like olive or coconut oil.

To go Keto, you'll need to cut out sugars, starchy vegetables and fruits, together with grains. Any diet should be discussed with a doctor before starting, but a ketogenic diet can be a great way for people to lose weight.

If you're tempted to cheat too much, you'll force their body out of ketosis, and it can be challenging to have to start over.

If you're keen to lose weight quickly, trying a Keto Mediterranean diet could be the way to go, for just a week or two, to jump start your weight loss.

During that time, you can start planning all the delicious foods you're going to include in your meal plan, as you move to the full Mediterranean diet and lifestyle.

7

TEN TIPS FOR SUCCESS

You now have a understanding of what it takes to become healthier by following a Mediterranean lifestyle.

Whether you're doing it because you want to lose weight, reduce depression symptoms, prevent cancer, or simply be happier overall, there are some core values for what is needed to do any of these.

Here's my ten tips to help you really make a success of moving towards a Mediterranean diet and lifestyle.

This is a refresher of what you've already learned, but it's time to turn your knowledge into action, so let's just recap some of the key points needed for success.

Plan Your Meals

Planning meals can be challenging. It's much easier to just go through a drive thru or pick out whatever's closest to the checkout line at the convenience store. You'll have to change the way you think to fully embrace the Mediterranean lifestyle.

It's time to plan your meals, as this can help to ensure that what you're going to be eating has all the proper nutrition that you need.

We've made it easy for you to get started, by including a 14-day meal plan, together with all the recipes you need, in the next chapter. Once you start planning your meals, it gets easier each week.

The key to starting is the knowledge you will have after you finish this book, as well as creating a well-stocked pantry that will make grocery shopping easier each week.

Having a full pantry will help make sure that you never put yourself in a position in which eating healthy isn't an option.

A solid pantry allows you to focus your money and shopping on getting foods that will help create meals that will include things you already have.

If you have a nice stock of pasta in your pantry, you can focus on just getting meat and vegetables at the store that week.

Having a variety of nuts, dried fruit, and seeds in the store cupboard will allow you to create whatever kind of salad you want.

Think of your pantry like your wardrobe. You wouldn't want to only have shirts that had specific matching pants, right? Keeping your pantry full of a variety of foods, means you need never get bored with your food!

Enjoy Your Food

This is a vital part of the Mediterranean lifestyle. If you're not enjoying your food, there's something wrong!

Make time to sit down each day and have a moment of peace while eating. Whether you do this with your family, or just with your friends, maybe even your pets, you need to make sure that you're enjoying mealtime and not just looking at it as a way to fill your stomach.

Focus on savoring every bite. Appreciate the fresh and delicious food that you get to eat. When you start caring about your meals, you'll find it's easier to build something delicious that doesn't make it feel like you're on a diet.

This is an important part of self-care as well. So often we'll just go and get some fast food, come home and shovel it in, and then end up feeling bad, either because of low self-esteem or just physically ill from the processed foods.

When you take the time to cook a meal, and then savor that meal, you're likely to feel much better about yourself afterwards.

A few people seem to be natural cooks, but there are plenty of other folks that have had to learn how to get better at preparing dishes.

Don't be afraid of the kitchen. It'll take practice to learn new recipes, but, as my gran always used to say, 'practice makes perfect!'.

Wherever your skills are at, you can learn to cook new recipes and you can definitely improve your culinary skills!

Schedule in Times of Relaxation

Taking time to relax is an intrinsic part of living a healthy lifestyle.

Don't you deserve to have some relaxation time?

It might be hard at first, especially for parents. Finding time to relax is important, if you're really wanting to improve your overall health and wellbeing.

This includes taking time to unplug from your phone. Some people might think that it's relaxing to play games for hours, but this probably isn't going to help make you feel better in the long run. Try to take time each day to shut your phone off, in order to rest and relax.

Some of us feel like they're being unproductive if they indulge in moments of self-care. We're always looking after others but we fail to look after ourselves.

That kind of thinking has to end. It is productive to relax. Consider it like re-charging your batteries. You return refreshed and ready for whatever life brings each day.

Remember, this is a diet that's about your lifestyle, as well as the food that you eat.

Taking time out for you, to do things you enjoy, is a vital part of living the Mediterranean lifestyle

Get Outside More

We've stressed the importance of getting outside to get some sun, but it's about far more than that.

Go for a walk and explore the things around you. Get a sense of yourself and what you enjoy by spending some time enjoying this beautiful world.

Get outside - feel the fresh air enter your lungs. Feel the sun hit your skin.

If you have the room and the weather permits, try eating outside as much as possible as well. You're just going to be sitting in a chair relaxing while you eat, so you may as well do it outside.

We all know that there's something re-energizing about being outside, we just have to get into the habit of doing it more often!

Eat Fresh Foods

Fresh food not only tastes better, but there's a plethora of health benefits that come along with those that eat fresh foods daily.

While it might be harder and more expensive to get hold of fresh food, it should still be done as often as possible.

Once you build your pantry, you'll start to realize that it's easier to create meals. You'll discover that the flavors of fresh food, are so superior to store bought staples. Not to mention, having the sense of accomplishment, that comes from having cooked your meal yourself!

Drink Plenty of Water

With so many different drinks available, few of us often drink water.

But the benefits of drinking water at the beginning of the day are clear. It helps to hydrate and cleanse the body. As you increase your water consumption, you'll see the benefit in how your hair and skin look and feel.

If you don't like the taste of water, keep a bottle in the fridge, or add a slice of lemon.

To make sure that you're getting plenty of water, invest in a   water bottle that you can carry around with you. Keep bottles filled with water in the fridge, so you always have something fresh and cold to drink.

Try to remember to drink enough water each day!

Practice Mindfulness

Mindfulness is all about becoming aware of one's surroundings, in order to escape our worries over the future and regrets about the past.

Become more aware of what's going on around you. Live each moment fully, instead of just moving through life as fast as you can.

Being mindful involves looking at all the things around you and grounding yourself in that moment.

Cut Out Sugar

Sugar tastes great and can be addictive. Sugar is not good for our health.

Cutting out sugar can be hard at first, probably because you're addicted to it.

Sugar is hidden in all sorts of foods, as well as being in some of our favorite naughty treats, such as ice cream and candy.

Be prepared for when those cravings start and have some tasty treats on hand. If you crave ice cream, try loading up on strawberries instead. If you need some chocolate or candy, eat some of your favorite nuts.

By cutting out sugar completely, you'll reduce those cravings within just a few days and find it easier to go without.

Spend Time with Loved Ones

The reason why people in the Mediterranean are so happy and healthy is that they put an emphasis on hanging out with friends and family.

You may not be physically or emotionally close to your biological family. If that's you, remember that friends are the family we choose for ourselves.

One of the easiest ways to spend time with those we love, is by sharing a meal together.

However you choose to spend time with your friends and family, choose to be fully present in the moment, so that you gain the most benefit from your time together.

Eat As Much As You Want

The best part of a Mediterranean diet is that there's no counting calories.

You don't have to weigh out your meals before you eat them. It's easy to remember what foods you can eat and what foods you should avoid. All you need to do is learn to listen to your body and you can eat as much as you want!

One of the main reasons why Mediterranean diet is so successful is because you don't have to worry about cutting down on how much you eat.   That means it's a diet you can stick to, for life!

LISA SCOTT

8

THE 14-DAY MEDITERRANEAN DIET MENU PLAN WITH RECIPES

To get you started, here's a 14-day menu plan, together with the recipes you'll need.

Once you've gotten started, you can start finding meals that are a good fit for the diet, and create your own plan, going forward.

Each of these recipes is for two people, unless otherwise stated.

Day 1

Breakfast: Herbed Omelette with Spinach and Feta

Lunch: Spicy Chickpea Salad with Greens

Snack: Crunchy Vegetable Wraps

Dinner: Instant Pot Mediterranean Chicken Casserole

Dessert: Strawberry Smoothie Cups

Day 2

Breakfast: Poached Eggs in Spicy Tomato Sauce

Lunch: Grilled Lemon Chicken with Parmesan Tomato

Snack: Handful of Unsalted Mixed Nuts

Dinner: Eggplant Parmesan

Dessert: Instant Pot Chocolate Pudding

Day 3

Breakfast: Blueberry Yogurt with Walnuts

Lunch: Steamed Vegetable Mix

Snack: Caprese Salad

Dinner: Italian Hasselback Chicken

Dessert: Roasted Honeyed Almonds

Day 4

Breakfast: Italian Frittata with Cherry Tomatoes

Lunch: Avocado Salad with Smoked Salmon

Snack: Mixed Berries with a dollop of Greek Yogurt

Dinner: Tuscan Style Salmon

Dessert: Watermelon Sorbet

Day 5

Breakfast: Egg Stuffed Bell Peppers

Lunch: Shrimp and Summer Veggie Bowl

Snack: Chili Roasted Chickpeas

Dinner: Skillet Garlic Chicken with Broccoli

Dessert: Fig and Cherry Bites

Day 6

Breakfast: Berry Cinnamon Oats

Lunch: Cauliflower Pizza Crust

Snack: Sweet Potato Wedges

Dinner: Cajun Chicken Lettuce Wraps

Dessert: Raspberry Frozen Yogurt

Day 7

Breakfast: Hash brown Casserole

Lunch: Lemon Parsley Pan Salmon

Snack: Parmesan Zucchini Sticks

Dinner: Instant Pot Stuffed Chicken

Dessert: Strawberry Cheesecake

Day 8

Breakfast: Tuscan Mini Quiche

Lunch: Crispy Feta with Egg Plant Ribbons

Snack: Instant Pot Savoury Cauliflower Fritters

Dinner: Seafood Stew

Dessert: Greek Yogurt Chocolate Mousse

Day 9

Breakfast: Breakfast Avocado Salad

Lunch: Arugula and Pine Nut Salad with Feta

Snack: Grapefruit Juice

Dinner: Creamy Chili Shrimp

Dessert: Coconut Cashew Bars

Day 10

Breakfast: Eggs with Tomato, Olives and Feta

Lunch: Balsamic Glazed Caprese Chicken

Snack: Mediterranean Feta Stuffed Bell Peppers

Dinner: Sweet Peppercorn Salmon

Dessert: No Bake Fruit Tart

Day 11

Breakfast: Fruit and Nut Yogurt

Lunch: Tomato Cucumber Salad with Olives and Feta

Snack: Kiwi Slices

Dinner: Stuffed Zucchini Boats

Dessert: Poached Pears with Walnuts

Day 12

Breakfast: Zucchini and Tomato Frittata

Lunch: Grilled Chicken Skewers

Snack: Strawberry Smoothie

Dinner: Eggplant Hasselback

Dessert: Cashew Cream Stuffed Strawberries

Day 13

Breakfast: Egg White Scramble with Spinach and Tomato

Lunch: Avocado Cucumber Chickpea Salad

Snack: Caprese Style Portobellos

Dinner: Tuscan Skillet Chicken

Dessert: Goat Cheese and Pistachio Stuffed Figs

Day 14

Breakfast: Crumbly Berry Breakfast Bake

Lunch: Crispy Parmesan Chicken with Vegetables

Snack: Herb Roasted Red Potatoes

Dinner: Garlic Lemon Salmon

Dessert: Apricot Energy Bites

Herbed Omelette with Spinach and Feta

Ingredients

>4 Eggs
>
>1 cup baby Spinach, chopped
>
>3 tbsp. Feta Cheese, cubed
>
>1 tbsp. Olive Oil
>
>½ tsp. Chives, thinly sliced
>
>½ tsp. Tarragon Leaves, finely chopped
>
>A few sprigs of Parsley
>
>1 tsp. Peppercorn, coarsely ground
>
>Salt, to taste

Preparation

- In a mixing bowl, combine eggs, spinach, chives, tarragon and parsley, and beat well.
- Season egg mixture with salt and pepper.

- Heat olive oil in a non-stick pan. Spread the eggs evenly in the pan.

- When the omelette has cooked from the bottom, add feta cheese to the top and gently flip.

- Remove omelette from the pan when completely cooked.

Spicy Chickpea Salad with Greens

Ingredients

1 15 oz. can Chickpeas, drained

2 cups Mixed Greens

1 large Cucumber, chopped

2 tbsp. Olive Oil

1 tbsp. Lime Juice

1/2 tsp. Paprika powder

Salt and black Pepper to taste

Preparation

- To prepare dressing, combine olive oil, lime juice and spices in a bowl.

- Toss greens, chickpeas and cucumbers together with the dressing and serve.

Crunchy Vegetable Wraps

Ingredients

1 head Iceberg Lettuce

½ cup Ricotta Cheese

½ cup Avocado Slices

1 Cucumber

4 Celery Stalks

1 Jalapeno Pepper

1 tbsp. Garlic, minced

Salt and Pepper, to taste

Preparation

- Julienne cucumbers and celery stalks into about 2-inch-long strips.

- Carefully wash each leaf of the lettuce and lay them out on individual parchment papers. Spread about 2 tablespoons of ricotta cheese on each leaf.

- Layer one lettuce leaf on top of the other and place cucumbers, celery, avocado and jalapenos on top. Season with salt and pepper.

- Carefully roll each lettuce leaf into a wrap and secure with a toothpick.

Instant Pot Mediterranean Chicken Casserole

Ingredients

1 lb. boneless, skinless Chicken thighs

1 Onion, chopped

1/3 cup Red Wine

16 oz. can Chopped Tomatoes

16 oz. bag frozen Mixed Vegetables

½ cup Black Olives

2 tbsp. Olive Oil

2 teaspoons Dried Parsley

2 teaspoons Dried Oregano

1 tsp. Paprika Powder

1 tsp. Onion Powder

Salt and black Pepper to taste

Preparation

- Select Sauté option on Instant Pot.

- Heat oil in the Instant Pot. Add chicken and let brown on both sides.

- Remove chicken and add onions. Cook until soft, for about 5 minutes.

- Add tomatoes, herbs and spices and cook for an additional 2-3 minutes.

- Add wine, frozen vegetables and the browned chicken. Mix well.

- Set Instant Pot to manual for about 8 minutes.

- Release steam. Add black olives, mix well and serve.

Strawberry Smoothie Cups

Ingredients

1 cup full fat Yogurt

1 cup frozen Strawberries

1 tsp. Honey

¼ tsp. Lemon Juice

½ cup Almonds, roughly chopped

Preparation

- Combine yogurt, strawberries, honey and lemon juice in a blender.

- Blend until smooth and creamy.

- Divide between two small bowls.

- Garnish with almond and serve.

Poached Eggs in Spicy Tomato Sauce

Ingredients

1 28 oz. Can of Chopped Tomatoes

4 Large Eggs

¼ cup Water

3 tbsp. Olive Oil

1 Small Onion, Finely Chopped

3 Large Cloves Garlic, Finely Chopped

1 tsp. Ground Coriander

2 tsp. Smoked Paprika

1/2 tsp. Salt

1/4 tsp. Black Pepper

2 to 3 tbsp. Fresh Parsley, Chopped

Preparation

- In a large skillet, heat olive oil and sauté onions until soft.

- Add chopped garlic and cook for 2 minutes.

- Add chopped tomatoes and cook for 10 to 15 minutes or until the sauce starts to thicken.

- Then add all the spices while continuing to stir.

- Add water to the sauce, mix and allow the sauce to simmer.

- Crack the eggs on top of the sauce and cover with a lid for about 5-7 minutes. Cook for an additional 2 minutes if you prefer a hard yolk.

- Once the eggs are done, remove from heat and garnish with fresh parsley.

- Serve hot.

Grilled Lemon Chicken with Parmesan Tomato

Ingredients

1 lb. Boneless Chicken Breast

2 tbsp. Lemon Juice, Freshly Squeezed

½ cup Extra Virgin Olive Oil

½ tsp. Salt

½ tsp. Ground Black Pepper

¼ tsp Garlic Powder

1 Large Tomato

¼ tsp. Oregano

¼ cup Parmesan Cheese, Grated

Preparation

- Add lemon juice, olive oil, salt, pepper and garlic powder to a shallow bowl. Mix vigorously to form a dressing.

- Cut each chicken breast in half so there are 4 even pieces. Marinated the chicken in the dressing for at least 30 minutes. Flip halfway through.

- Grill for 5 to 7 minutes each side or bake on 400F for 25-30 minutes or until the chicken is cooked through and golden brown.

- Cut the tomato in half and place on a baking sheet cut side up. Sprinkle with salt, pepper and oregano. Cover with parmesan cheese and drizzle olive oil on top.

- Bake for 20 minutes on 400F or until the cheese is melted with a golden top.

Eggplant Parmesan

Ingredients

1 pound Eggplant (about 2 small)

1/8 cup Olive Oil + 2 tbsp., divided

1 small yellow Onion, finely Chopped

2 cloves Garlic, minced

1/8 cup Tomato Sauce

1 14 oz. can of Crushed Tomatoes

¼ cup freshly chopped Fresh Basil

½ tsp. Balsamic Vinegar

Pinch of Red Pepper Flakes

Salt, to taste

1 cup freshly grated Mozzarella Cheese

½ cup freshly grated Parmesan Cheese

Preparation

- Preheat oven to 425F and line one large baking sheet with parchment paper.

- Slice off rounded ends of the eggplants and slice length wise to make long even slabs.

- Brush the eggplants with olive oil and sprinkle with salt and pepper. Arrange in a single layer on the baking sheet.

- Roast for about 20 minutes or until golden and tender. Set aside.

- Meanwhile, heat the 2 tbsp. olive oil and sauté the onions until tender.

- Add garlic and tomato sauce. Cook for 1 minute while stirring. Add crushed tomatoes and stir.

- Simmer for 15 minutes on low heat until the sauce has thickened.

- Remove from heat and add chopped basil, vinegar, salt and red pepper flakes.

- In the bottom of a baking dish, spread sauce until it covers the bottom.

- Arrange the roasted eggplant on top. Spoon some sauce over it and spread half the mozzarella cheese.

- Arrange rest of the eggplant on the cheese layer and top with sauce and the remaining mozzarella.

- Evenly sprinkle parmesan on top and bake uncovered for about 15-20 minutes until the top is golden and the sauce bubbles.

- Cool for 15 minutes before serving. Garnish with fresh basil leaves.

Instant Pot Chocolate Pudding

Ingredients

      2 cups 2% Milk

      4 Egg Yolks

      ¼ cup Cocoa Powder

      ¼ cup unsweetened Cooking Chocolate

      ¾ teaspoon Concentrated Stevia Extract

      a drop of Vanilla Essence

      Pinch of Salt

Preparation

- In the Instant Pot, heat milk until it begins to simmer.
- Remove from heat. Chop cooking chocolate and mix until melted.
- In a separate bowl, whisk together egg yolks, stevia, cocoa powder, vanilla and salt until well combined.
- Add the egg mixture into the chocolate mixture until blended together uniformly.
- Strain and pour into a 6 inch round baking dish. Cover tightly with aluminium foil.
- Add 1½ cup of water into the Instant pot and place the baking dish on the trivet. Cook on low pressure for about 22 minutes. Naturally release pressure.
- Uncover the dish and let it cool. Refrigerate for 3-4 hours before serving.

Blueberry Yogurt with Walnuts

Ingredients

> 2 cups Greek Yogurt
>
> 1½ cup Blueberries
>
> 3 tbsp. Walnuts, chopped

Preparation

- Combine yogurts and blueberries in a bowl. Mix together.
- Top with walnuts and serve.

Steamed Vegetable Mix

Ingredients

> ½ cup Peas
>
> 1 large Potato, Cut into Cubes
>
> 1 large Carrot, Slices
>
> 1 head Broccoli, cut into bite sized pieces
>
> ½ lb. Green Beans
>
> 2 tbsp. Olive Oil
>
> 1 tbsp. Lemon Juice
>
> ½ tsp. Salt
>
> 1 tsp. Black Pepper

Preparation

- In a large pot, add all the vegetables and toss with salt, pepper, lemon juice and olive oil.
- Add half a cup of water and put on high heat.
- When steam forms, lower the heat to simmer and cover with lid.
- Cook for 20-25 minutes or until the vegetables are tender.

Caprese Salad

Ingredients

2 large ripe Tomatoes

½ lb Buffalo Mozzarella, cut into ¼ inch thick slices

½ cup Basil Leaves

¼ tsp. Salt

¼ tsp. Black Pepper

2 tbsp. Olive Oil

1 tsp. Vinegar

Preparation

- Arrange tomato slices on a serving plate. Sprinkle salt on top.
- Insert mozzarella slices between the sliced tomatoes.
- Garnish with fresh basil leaves and sprinkle black pepper on top.
- Drizzle with olive oil and vinegar.
- Let sit in the refrigerator for 20 minutes and serve.

Italian Hasselback Chicken

Ingredients

2 Boneless Skinless Chicken Breast Halves

¼ cup Sun Dried Tomatoes

1/2 cup Mozzarella Cheese, Cut into Strips

½ cup Mushrooms, Slices

¼ cup Fresh Basil Leaves

1 tbsp. Lemon Juice, Freshly Squeezed

¼ cup Extra Virgin Olive Oil

¼ tsp. Salt

¼ tsp. Oregano

¼ tsp. Mixed Herbs

Preparation

- Preheat oven to 350F.

- On tops of the chicken breast halves, make slices from top to almost bottom and 3/4-inch apart to form pockets; be sure not to cut all the way through.

- Add lemon juice, olive oil, salt, oregano and herbs to a bowl and mix. Rub onto the chicken breasts, including the pockets.

- Combine mushrooms and sun dried tomatoes and place on bottom of a glass baking dish.

- Place chicken breasts on top of the mushroom tomato base.

- Insert slices of Mozzarella cheese in the pockets cut into the chicken breasts. Bake for

30 minutes or until the chicken is cooked through.

- Garnish with fresh basil leaves

Roasted Honeyed Almonds

Ingredients

¼ cup Almonds

3 tbsp. Honey

1 tbsp. Sesame Seeds

Preparation

- Boil a pot of water and add in the almonds, boiling for 60 seconds
- Drain the water over a strainer and rinse under cold water to cool quickly
- Pinch the ends to remove the skins off the almonds.
- Pat dry with a paper towel.
- Place the almonds and honey into a saucepan and place over a medium to low heat.
- Cook until the almonds are slightly golden and remove from the heat
- Pour the honey and almond mixture into bowls and finish off with a sprinkle of sesame seeds
- Allow to cool before serving.

Italian Frittata with Cherry Tomatoes

Ingredients

> 4 Eggs
>
> 1 cup Cherry Tomatoes
>
> ½ cup Mushrooms
>
> ½ cup Artichoke hearts, drained and chopped
>
> ½ cup Mozzarella Cheese
>
> ¼ cup Full Fat Milk
>
> 2 Green Onions, Chopped
>
> 1 Clove of Garlic, Minced
>
> 2 tbsp. Olive Oil
>
> 1 tsp. Mixed Herbs
>
> Salt, to taste
>
> Pepper, to taste

Preparation

- Dice mushrooms and chop cherry tomatoes finely.

- Heat olive oil and sauté garlic for one minute. Then add green onions, artichoke hearts, mushrooms and cherry tomatoes.

- Whisk the eggs and add milk, cheese, herbs and the sautéed vegetables. Add salt and pepper according to your liking and mix well.

- Grease a 6-inch baking pan and pour the mixture in it.

- • Bake in a preheated oven until the eggs are cooked through and cheese melted.

Avocado Salad with Smoked Salmon

Ingredients

50 g Smoked Salmon

1 Pear, Sliced

1 red Onion, finely sliced

1 cup Rocket

1 Avocado, peeled & sliced

2 Cherry Tomatoes, sliced

2 tbsp Olive oil

Juice of 1 Lemon

Salt and pepper, to taste

½ bunch parsley, to garnish

Preparation

- To prepare dressing, combine olive oil, lemon juice, salt and pepper in a bowl.
- Gently toss the salad ingredients with the dressing and serve immediately.

Tuscan Style Salmon

Ingredients

2 6 oz. Salmon Fillets

2 cups Grape Tomatoes

1 cup Green Beans

4 Large Cloves of Garlic, crushed

¼ cup Fresh Parsley, chopped

¼ cup Lemon Juice

4 tbsp. Olive Oil

1 tbsp. Lemon Zest

¼ tsp. Salt

¼ tsp. Black Pepper, freshly ground

Preparation

- Preheat oven to 400 degrees F. Use nonstick spray to coat a large baking sheet.

- Place salmon fillets in the middle of the baking sheet.

- Mix half the olive oil with garlic, parsley, lemon juice, zest, salt and pepper. Spread this mixture on top of the salmon fillets.

- Toss green beans and tomatoes with the rest of the olive oil and season with salt and pepper.

- Arrange beans and tomatoes around the salmon and bake for about 20 minutes or until the fish is flaky.

- Let rest for 3 minutes and serve.

Egg Stuffed Bell Pepper

Ingredients

2 Eggs

1 large Bell Pepper

½ cup shredded Cheddar Cheese

¼ cup chopped Spinach Leaves

2 tbsp. Chopped Black Olives

A pinch of Tarragon

Black Pepper, to taste

Salt, to taste

Preparation

- Preheat oven to 400F.
- Cut bell peppers width wise and remove the seeds.
- Place peppers on a baking sheet and bake for 5 minutes
- In a mixing bowl, combine eggs, spinach, olives, tarragon, salt and pepper and beat well.
- Spoon egg mixture into the bell peppers and top with cheese.
- Bake for 20 minutes or until the eggs are set.
- Serve immediately.

Shrimp and Summer Veggie Bowl

Ingredients

½ lb. Shrimp, without tails

1 tsp. minced Ginger

1 tsp. Lime juice

2 tbsp. Olive oil

½ tsp. Garlic powder

½ tsp. Paprika powder

½ tsp. Onion powder

1 medium Zucchini, cut into quarters lengthwise

1 small Bell Pepper, cut into squares

½ cup Corn kernels

Salt and pepper, to taste

¼ cup fresh Parsley

Preparation

- Combine lime juice with all the spices. Add in the shrimp and toss well to coat.

- In a large skillet, heat olive oil and toss in shrimp. Add in the vegetables as well.

- Cook for 5-7 minutes or until the shrimp is no longer pink and the vegetables are tender.

- Garnish with fresh parsley.

Chili Roasted Chickpeas

Ingredients

1 15 oz. can Chickpeas, drained

1 tbsp. Olive oil

½ tbsp. Chili Powder

¼ tbsp. Salt

½ tsp Smoked Paprika

½ tsp. Garlic powder

¼ tsp. Black Pepper

Preparation

- Preheat oven to 400F.

- Pat dry the chickpeas using paper towels.

- In a bowl, mix the chickpeas with olive oil.

- Spray a baking sheet with non-stick cooking spray. Arrange the chickpeas in a single layer on the sheet.

- Bake for about 30 minutes or until nice and crisp, stirring halfway through.

- Combine the seasoning ingredients and toss in the roasted chickpeas.

Skillet Chicken with Broccoli and Mushrooms

Ingredients

1 lb. boneless Chicken breast fillets

1 cup chopped Broccoli

1 cup chopped Mushrooms

½ cup plain Greek Yogurt

½ cup Chicken broth

¼ cup Full Fat Milk

2 tbsp. Extra Virgin Olive Oil

1 tbsp. Cream Cheese

4-5 cloves Garlic, minced

½ tsp. Oregano

½ tsp. Mixed herbs

½ tsp. Salt

½ tsp. Ground Black Pepper

Preparation

- Mix together minced garlic, salt, pepper and yogurt. Rub onto the chicken and set aside for 10 minutes in the refrigerator.

- Heat olive oil in a skillet and add chicken fillets. Cook for about 2 minutes on each side on high heat or until the exterior of the chicken is golden brown.

- Lower the heat and add the broth and milk. Add oregano and mixed herbs. Cover with a lid and allow to cook on low heat for 10 minutes.

- Add in mushrooms and broccoli and bring to a simmer. Cook until the broccoli is tender. Add in cream cheese.

- When the sauce has thickened, remove from heat and serve.

Fig and Cherry Bites

Ingredients

10 dried Figs

½ cup dry Cherries

½ cup chopped Hazelnuts

¼ tsp. Cinnamon powder

½ tbsp. Maple syrup

½ cup shredded Coconut

Preparation

- In a food processor, pulse cherries and hazelnuts until very finely chopped.

- Place into a bowl and set aside.

- Now pulse together figs, cinnamon and maple syrup to form a paste.

- Add in the cherry mixture and pulse to combine.

- Transfer this mixture to a bowl and place in the freezer for 10 minutes. The chilled mixture is easier to form into balls. But this step can be skipped if short of time.

- Take 1 tbsp. of mixture and shape into a ball. Repeat until all the mixture is used up.

- Roll the balls in shredded coconut and serve.

Berry Cinnamon Oats

Ingredients

50 g Gluten Free Oats

¼ cup Water

¼ tsp. ground Cinnamon

½ cup Milk

½ cup Yogurt

1 cup Mixed Berries

½ tsp. Honey

Preparation

- In a small saucepan, add water and oats. Cook for 2 minutes on medium heat and bring to a boil.

- Add milk, cinnamon and honey, stirring constantly.

- Turn down the heat and transfer to a bowl.

- When the oats have slightly cooled, top with mixed berries and serve with a dollop of yogurt.

Cauliflower Pizza Crust

Ingredients

1 lb. frozen Cauliflower Florets

1 Egg

1 Bell Pepper, sliced

½ Onion, sliced

¼ cup sliced Black Olives

½ cup Pizza Sauce

½ cup grated Parmesan Cheese

1 cup Mozzarella Cheese

1 tsp. Mixed Herbs

1 tsp. Oregano

1/8 tsp. Salt

¼ tsp. Black Pepper

Preparation

- Thaw cauliflower florets completely.

- Pulse the florets in a food processor until it resembles a rice texture.

- Line a large bowl with cheesecloth and place cauliflower rice in it.

- Lift up the corners of the cheesecloth and squeeze out the moisture from the cauliflower to as much as possible.

- Use a kitchen towel to remove any remaining moisture.

- In a bowl, add the dry cauliflower rice, egg, parmesan, salt, pepper and mixed herbs. Mix well.

- Line a baking sheet with parchment paper. Spread this mixture on top of the paper in the shape of pizza crust.

- Bake in a preheated oven at 400F for 20 minutes.

- Top with pizza sauce, olives, onions, bell pepper and mozzarella. Sprinkle oregano on top.

- Bake for 10 more minutes or until the cheese is melted and golden.

Sweet Potato Wedges

Ingredients

2 large Sweet Potatoes

2 tbsp. Olive Oil

1 tbsp. Lime Juice

1/2 tsp. Paprika Powder

½ tsp. Garlic Powder

1 tsp. Salt

½ tsp. Black Pepper

Preparation

- Preheat oven to 400F and line a baking sheet with aluminium foil.

- Cut off the ends of the sweet potatoes and peel them (optional). Slice sweet potatoes into large wedges.

- In a large bowl, add olive oil, lime juice, paprika powder, garlic powder, salt and pepper. Add the wedges and toss well to combine.

- Arrange the wedges on the baking sheet in a single layer and bake for 30 minutes.

- Turn on broiler and cook for an additional 3 minutes.

- Cool slightly and serve.

Cajun Chicken Lettuce Wraps

Ingredients

6 large leaves Butter Lettuce

½ cup Cream Cheese

1 small Tomato, sliced

½ red Onion, sliced

3-4 fresh Basil leaves

1 tbsp. Pickled Peppers

1 tsp. Mustard

1 tsp, Cajun seasoning

4 boneless Chicken thighs, cut into strips

¼ cup Yogurt

2 tbsp. Olive oil

1 tbsp. Garlic, minced

Salt and Pepper, to taste

Preparation

- Marinate chicken strips in a mixture of yogurt, Cajun seasoning, garlic, salt and pepper for half an hour.
- Heat olive oil in a non-stick pan and cook chicken strips completely.
- Spread cream cheese and mustard on each lettuce leaf.
- Place chicken on top as well as pickled peppers, onion, tomato.
- Garnish with basil and serve.

Raspberry Frozen Yogurt

Ingredients

100 g Frozen Raspberries

1 cup Greek Yogurt

2 tbsp. Honey

Preparation

- Add all ingredients in a blender and blend until smooth and creamy.

- Scoop out into bowls and serve.

Hash Brown Casserole

Ingredients

1 1 lb. package frozen Hash Browns

1 can cream of Mushroom

½ cup Sour Cream

1 cup shredded Mozzarella Cheese

½ cup shredded Cheddar Cheese

1/2 tsp. Onion Powder

½ tsp. Garlic Powder

¼ tsp. Salt

½ tsp. Black Pepper

Preparation

- Preheat oven to 350F and spray a medium sized baking dish with non-stick spray.

- In a large bowl, combine hash browns, cream of mushroom, sour cream, mozzarella cheese along with all the seasonings.

- Mix well and pour into the baking dish.

- Top with shredded cheddar and bake for 30 minutes or so until done.

Lemon Parsley Pan Salmon

Ingredients

2 6 oz. Salmon Fillets, with skin

1 tsp. minced Garlic

¼ cup Fresh Parsley, chopped

1 tbsp. Lemon Juice

4 tbsp. Olive Oil

1 tsp. Lemon Zest

¼ tsp. Salt

¼ tsp. Black Pepper, freshly ground

Preparation

- Prepare salmon by drying the fillets on paper towels prior to cooking.
- Rub the fillets with a mixture of minced garlic, lemon zest, salt and pepper.
- Heat olive oil in a skillet and place the fillets in it, skin side down.
- Cook for about 5-6 minutes, if the fish does not release easily, wait a minute or two longer.
- Flip, and cook for an additional 3 minutes on the other side until the salmon is completely opaque and flakes easily.
- Sprinkle lemon juice on the fillets and garnish generously with parsley.

Parmesan Zucchini Sticks

Ingredients

2 Zucchinis, quartered lengthwise

1 tbsp. Olive oil

¼ cup Parmesan Cheese, grated

¼ tsp. dried Oregano

¼ tsp. dried Thyme

¼ tsp. Mixed Herbs

¼ cup freshly Chopped Fresh Basil

Salt, to taste

Pepper, to taste

Preparation

- Preheat oven to 350F and line one large baking sheet with parchment paper.
- Combine parmesan, oregano, thyme, mixed herbs, salt, pepper and olive oil in a bowl.
- Toss the zucchini sticks in the parmesan mixture and arrange in a single layer on the baking sheet.
- Bake for about 15 minutes, then broil for 2-3 minutes until golden and crisp.
- Garnish with fresh basil and serve.

Instant Pot Stuffed Chicken

Ingredients

2 Boneless Chicken Breasts

1 tsp. Lemon Juice

½ tsp. Garlic Powder

½ tsp. Paprika Powder

½ tsp. Mustard Powder

1 tbsp. Olive Oil

Salt, to taste

Black Pepper, to taste

For the Stuffing

½ cup Shredded Mozzarella Cheese

½ cup Shredded Cheddar Cheese

¼ cup Pitted Black Olives

Preparation

- In a bowl, mix lemon juice, garlic powder, paprika and mustard powder.

- Slit each chicken breast from the middle carefully.

- Rub the marinade on the chicken breasts and refrigerate for 2-4 hours at least.

- Mix the cheese and olives and stuff each breast with this mixture. Seal the breasts with toothpicks.

- Put olive oil in the pot and sauté chicken breasts for 3-4 minutes each side.

- Remove chicken breasts. Put 1 cup of water and place chicken on the trivet in the pot. Cook for 8 minutes. Release the pressure naturally and keep the lid on for an additional 10 minutes.

- Take the chicken breasts out of the Instant Pot, remove toothpicks and serve.

Strawberry Cheesecake

Ingredients

½ cup raw Almonds

½ cup raw Cashews

1 tbsp. Honey

1 cups fresh Strawberries

½ cup Strawberry Puree

¼ tsp. Lemon Juice

1 cup cream Cheese

¼ cup whipping Cream

Preparation

- Pulse nuts in a food processor until very finely chopped. Transfer to a bowl and mix thoroughly with honey.

- In a small spring form pan, press *down the* nut mixture to form a crust.

- Combine whipping cream, cream cheese, lemon juice and strawberry puree. Mix well and spoon on top of the crust.

- Garnish with fresh strawberries. Chill before serving.

Tuscan Mini Quiche

Ingredients

> 4 eggs, beaten
>
> 1 cup shredded Cheddar Cheese
>
> ¼ cup Spinach leaves, chopped
>
> ½ cup red pepper diced
>
> ¼ cup grape tomatoes, halved
>
> 1 tbsp. Olive Oil
>
> ½ tsp. Garlic Powder
>
> ¼ tsp. Salt
>
> ½ tsp. Black Pepper

Preparation

- Preheat oven to 400F and spray a muffin pan with non-stick spray.
- Mix together eggs with salt, pepper, garlic powder. Add in the chopped spinach and grape tomatoes.
- Pour this mixture into each cup until ¾ full.
- Top with shredded cheddar and bake for 15 minutes or so until done.

Crispy Feta with Eggplant Ribbons

Ingredients

> 6 oz. Feta Cheese

¼ cup Almond Flour

3+3 tbsp. Olive Oil

2 Eggplants

1 egg, beaten

1 oz. Green Olives, Pitted and Sliced

1 tbsp. Minced Garlic

1 tsp. Dried Basil

Preparation

- Cut feta cheese into thick cubes of about 2 inches. Dip the cheese cubes into the beaten egg, then dredge in almond flour and refrigerate.

- Heat oil in the Instant Pot on high, and fry the cubes for about a minute until they turn crisp.

- Place the crispy feta on paper towels and put aside.

- Wash eggplants, form noodles using spiralizer or cut into ribbons using a peeler.

- Place ½ cup water in the Pot. Add eggplant and cook in the Instant Pot for 2 minutes. Release pressure manually. Place cooked eggplant aside.

- Dry the Pot and heat oil. Sauté garlic and add the eggplant. Add olives and season with salt and pepper.

- Remove from heat and mix with the crispy feta.

- Sprinkle basil and drizzle olive oil on top.

Instant Pot Savoury Cauliflower Fritters

Ingredients

    1 Cauliflower

    ¼ cup Olive Oil

    ¼ cup Cheddar Cheese

    ¼ cup Mozzarella Cheese

    2 eggs

    1 Chilli Pepper, Finely Chopped

    ½ tsp. Garlic Powder

    Salt, to taste

    Pepper, to taste

Preparation

- Cut the cauliflower into small florets, removing leaves and cutting out core. Put 1 cup of water in the Instant pot and set florets on a steamer basket to be placed on top of the trivet. Cook for 5 minutes and release pressure immediately.

- Mash the steamed cauliflower and dry well with paper towels. Add the shredded cheeses, eggs, chilli, salt and pepper. Mix well and shape into slightly flat patties.

- Heat oil in the Instant Pot. Shallow fry the patties until they are crisp on both sides.

Seafood Stew

Ingredients

> 1 cup Chicken Stock
>
> 1 cup Coconut Milk
>
> ¼ lb. Shrimp
>
> ¼ lb. Mussels
>
> ¼ cup Coconut Cream
>
> 4 oz. Fish (Salmon or Halibut)
>
> 3 tbsp. Olive Oil
>
> 2 tbsp. Lemon Juice
>
> 2 cloves Garlic, Crushed
>
> ½ tsp. Black Pepper
>
> ¼ tsp. Salt

Preparation

- In the Instant Pot, sauté the garlic.
- Add stock and coconut milk. Rub lemon juice, salt and pepper on fish fillets and place in the Pot. Add shrimp and mussels as well.
- Cook for 10 minutes. Release pressure naturally.
- Add coconut cream and allow to simmer for 5 minutes.
- Serve warm.

Greek Yogurt Chocolate Mousse

Ingredients

>½ cup Milk
>
>50 g Dark Chocolate, finely chopped
>
>2 cups Greek Yogurt
>
>¼ tsp. Vanilla Extract

Preparation

- Add milk to a small saucepan and place on slow heat. Add the dark chocolate.
- Keep stirring with a spatula until the two ingredients are combined well. Keep the heat low.
- Add honey and vanilla extract and mix well.
- Remove from heat and cool.
- Mix the chocolate milk with the Greek yogurt and transfer to individual ramekins or bowls.
- Chill for at least 2 hours in the refrigerator. Top with a dollop of Greek yogurt and fresh strawberries. Serve.

Breakfast Avocado Salad

Ingredients

>2 Eggs
>
>1 Boneless Chicken Thigh, cut into strips

2 cups Baby Greens

4 Cherry Tomatoes, quartered

1 Avocado, diced

1 tbsp. Olive Oil

1 tbsp. Apple Cider Vinegar

¼ tsp. Salt

½ tsp. Black Pepper

Preparation

- In a small pan, heat olive oil and add the chicken. Cook on medium heat until done.

- Poach the eggs and season with salt and pepper.

- In a large bowl, combine the baby greens, grape tomatoes, avocado, cooked chicken and apple cider vinegar.

- Top with the poached eggs and serve.

Arugula Salad with Pine Nuts and Feta

Ingredients

3 tbsp. Pine Nuts

1 bunch Arugula, thick stems discarded

1 large head Iceberg Lettuce, cut in half then sliced thinly

¼ cup Feta Cheese

¼ cup Grape Tomatoes, halved

1 tbsp. Lemon juice, freshly squeezed

2 tbsp. Olive Oil

Salt and pepper, to taste

¼ cup fresh Parsley

Preparation

- Combine lemon juice with olive oil, salt and pepper.
- Add the lettuce, arugula, pine nuts, feta cheese and grape tomatoes.
- Toss well and serve.

Creamy Chili Shrimp

Ingredients

1 lb. shrimp

½ Bell Pepper, cut into thin strips

½ cup White Cabbage, shredded

½ cup Chicken Stock

3 tbsp. Olive Oil

1 tbsp. Heavy Cream

1 Green Chilli

1 tbsp. Garlic, minced

1 tbsp. Ginger, cut into thin long strips

½ tsp. Cayenne Powder

½ tsp. Black Pepper

½ tsp. Lime Juice

Preparation

- Deseed and cut the green chilli into thin strips lengthwise.

- In the Instant Pot, sauté the bell pepper, cabbage and green chilli with half oil for 3-4 minutes. Remove and keep warm by covering with foil.

- Sautee ginger and garlic in the Instant Pot with the rest of the oil and add shrimp.

- Turn off sauté function. Add the spices and lime juice.

- Add chicken stock and cook on high pressure for 4 minutes.

- Release steam, add the sautéed vegetables and mix well.

- Add heavy cream and sauté until the sauce thickens slightly. Serve.

Coconut Cashew Bars

Ingredients

1 cup Raw Cashews

1 tbsp. Honey

½ cup Dried Apricots

½ cup Shredded Coconut

1 tbsp. Milk

½ tsp. Vanilla Extract

Preparation

- Soak dried apricots in very hot water for 15 minutes. Drain and then pulse along with cashews in a food processor until very finely chopped.

- Transfer to a bowl and mix thoroughly with honey, shredded coconut, milk and vanilla extract.

- Line a baking dish with parchment paper. Press down this mixture evenly into the dish.

- Refrigerate for at least 1 hour.

- Lift the parchment paper and place onto a cutting board. Cut into small bars. Serve.

Baked Eggs with Tomatoes, Olives and Feta

Ingredients

3 Eggs

100g Feta Cheese

½ can of Diced Tomatoes

¼ cup Cherry Tomatoes

¼ cup Green Olives

3 cloves of Garlic, crushed

2 tbsp. Olive Oil

1 tsp. Oregano

¼ tsp. Salt

½ tsp. Black Pepper

Preparation

- Sauté the garlic in olive oil. Add the tomatoes and oregano. Cook for 10 minutes and season with salt and pepper.

- In a baking dish, arrange the feta, olives and cherry tomatoes. Top with the cooked tomatoes.

- Preheat oven to 350F. Bake for 15 minutes.

- Remove from oven and crack the eggs on top. Cover with foil and turn the heat to 400F.

- Bake for 10 more minutes or until the eggs are done. Serve.

Balsamic Glazed Caprese Chicken

Ingredients

1 lb. Boneless Chicken Thighs

1 cup Cherry Tomatoes, halved

6 oz. Fresh Mozzarella, cut into 4 even slices

2 tbsp. minced Red Onion

¼ cup Balsamic Vinegar

¼ cup Red Wine

1 tsp. Honey

½ tsp. Mustard

6-8 fresh Basil leaves

2 tbsp. Olive oil

2 tbsp. Garlic, minced

Salt and Pepper, to taste

Preparation

- Season chicken thighs with salt and pepper.

- Heat a large skillet and add olive oil. Sauté garlic and onion.

- Add the chicken thighs and cook on both sides, at least 5 minutes each side until cooked though.

- Remove the chicken. Add the balsamic vinegar, wine, honey and mustard to the skillet.

- Constantly stir using a whisk. Allow it to simmer for 5 minutes.

- Add the chicken to the skillet and spoon the glaze on top.

- Add the mozzarella slices on top of the chicken. Cover and cook on low for 3-5 minutes or until the cheese is melted.

- Remove from heat.

- Garnish with cherry tomatoes and basil. Serve while hot.

Mediterranean Stuffed Peppers

Ingredients

2 Bell Peppers

½ cup Feta Cheese

3 tbsp. Greek Yogurt

1 clove Garlic, minced

1 tsp. Lemon Juice

1 tsp. Olive Oil

¼ tsp. Salt

Chopped Parsley, for garnishing

Preparation

- Preheat oven to 400F.

- Line a baking sheet with parchment paper.

- Slice in half and remove seeds and stems from the bell pepper.

- Place the peppers, sliced side down on the baking sheet.

- Roast for 15 minutes or less, removing when the peppers begin to char.

- Combine and feta and yogurt in a small bowl with salt and garlic.

- Stuff the roasted peppers with this mixture. Top with lemon juice and olive oil.

- Garnish with parsley and serve immediately.

Sweet Peppercorn Salmon

Ingredients

2 Salmon Fillets

2 tbsp. Olive Oil

2 tbsp. Parsley

1 tsp. Lemon Juice

1 tsp. Soya Sauce

1 tsp. Apple Cider Vinegar

½ tsp. Peppercorn, coarsely ground

½ tsp. Minced Ginger

Salt, to taste

1 tsp. Honey

Preparation

- Select the Sauté option on the Instant Pot and add butter, ginger, honey, lemon juice, vinegar, soy sauce. Cook for about a minute.

- Rub the salmon fillets with salt and pepper and place inside the Instant Pot. Spoon sauce over the fillets. Add 1/8 cup water and cook on low pressure for 1 minute.

- Release pressure manually. Flip with care and sauté salmon until cooked to your liking.

- Take out salmon from the pot and let the sauce simmer for an additional 3 to 4 minutes.

- Drizzle sauce over the fillets and garnish with parsley.

No Bake Fruit Tart

Ingredients

1 cup Almond Meal

¼ cup Unsweetened Cocoa Powder

2 tbsp. Maple Syrup

1 cup Greek Yogurt

4 oz. Bittersweet Chocolate, finely chopped

1 cup Mixed Berries

Preparation

- Combine almond meal with maple syrup and cocoa powder and mix well. Press down this mixture into 2 individual mini tart pans to form a crust.

- Melt the chocolate in a double boiler. Cool slightly and mix with the Greek yogurt.

- Pour this filling into the tart crusts. Top with mixed berries. Serve chilled.

Fruit and Nut Yogurt

Ingredients

> 1 cup Vanilla Yogurt
>
> ½ cup Strawberries
>
> ½ cup Raspberries
>
> 2 tbsp. Sunflower Seeds
>
> 2 tbsp. Pumpkin Seeds
>
> 6 tbsp. Unsalted Mixed Nuts, chopped

Preparation

- Mix the seeds, yogurt and berries.
- Top with nuts. Serve.

Tomato Cucumber Salad with Feta and Olives

Ingredients

> 1 cup Grape Tomatoes, cut in half
>
> 1 large Cucumber, diced
>
> ¼ cup Feta Cheese
>
> ¼ cup Kalamata Olives, drained, pitted and sliced
>
> 1 tbsp. Olive Oil
>
> 1 tbsp. Red Wine Vinegar

1 tsp. fresh Dill

½ tsp. Dried Oregano

1/8 tsp. Salt

Preparation

- Prepare dressing by whisking together olive oil, red wine vinegar, oregano and salt.
- In a large bowl, combine salad ingredients such as grape tomatoes, cucumber, olives and feta cheese.
- Toss the ingredients with the prepared dressing.
- Garnish with fresh dill and serve.

Stuffed Zucchini Boats

Ingredients

2 Zucchinis

1 cup cooked shredded Chicken

½ cup Feta Cheese

½ cup finely chopped Cucumber

¼ cup Black Olives, drained, pitted and sliced

1 tbsp. Olive Oil

1 tbsp. Red Wine Vinegar

1 tsp. Lemon Juice

½ tsp. Dried Oregano

1/8 tsp. Salt

Preparation

- Preheat oven to 350F.

- Prepare zucchinis by cutting lengthwise and scooping out the insides to form hollow boats.

- Place in a shallow baking dish and drizzle with olive oil.

- Bake for 12-15 minutes or until tender.

- Mix the chick**en, feta chee**se, cucumber and olives. Add red wine vinegar, lemon juice, oregano and salt.

- Top with more feta cheese and broil for about 2-3 minutes.

Poached Pears with Walnuts

Ingredients

2 large ripe Pears

2 tsp. Honey

½ cup Crushed Walnuts

½ tsp. Ground Cinnamon

Preparation

- Preheat oven to 350F.

- Cut the pears in half and scoop out the seeds.

- Place cut side up on a baking sheet lined with parchment paper.

- Sprinkle ground cinnamon and then walnuts on top.

- Drizzle with honey.

- Bake in the oven for 30 minutes.

- Remove. Let cool slightly.

- Serve warm with a dollop of frozen yogurt.

Zucchini and Tomato Frittata

Ingredients

4 Eggs

½ cup shredded Mozzarella Cheese

¼ cup Tomatoes, chopped

¼ cup Red Pepper, diced

1 small Zucchini, sliced

1 tbsp. Olive Oil

½ tsp. Garlic Powder

1/8 tsp. Salt

½ tsp. Cayenne Pepper

Preparation

- Preheat oven to 400F.

- Heat oil in a skillet. Add the zucchini slices and cook until tender, turning periodically.

- Turn off the heat and add red peppers.

- Whisk eggs in a separate bowl, with salt, pepper and garlic powder.

- Add tomatoes to the skillet and add the egg mixture.

- Mix well and top with cheese.

- Bake for about 10 minutes or until the eggs are done.

- Cool and serve.

Grilled Chicken Skewers

Ingredients

½ lb. Boneless Chicken Breast, cubed

1 Red Onion, cut into 1 inch pieces

1 Red Bell Pepper, cut into 1 inch pieces

1 small Zucchini, cut into 1 inch pieces

2 tbsp. Honey

3 tbsp. Olive Oil

4 tbsp. Red Wine

½ tsp. Garlic, minced

Salt and Pepper, to taste

Preparation

- Whisk together olive oil, red wine, honey, garlic, salt and pepper.

- Add the chicken, bell peppers, zucchini and red onion to the marinade and toss well.

- Marinate in the refrigerator for 1-2 hours. In the meanwhile, soak wooden skewers in cold water for 30 minutes.

- Thread chicken and vegetables onto the skewers.

- Preheat broiler. Spray non-stick spray on sheet pan.

- Place skewers in a single layer on the sheet pan. Broil for 5-7 minutes.

- Flip the skewers and broil for another 5-7 minutes.

Strawberry Smoothie

Ingredients

1 cup 2% Milk

1 tbsp. Honey

1 cup Frozen Strawberries

½ cup Vanilla Yogurt

Preparation

- Place ingredients in a blender and cover with lid.

- Blend until smooth.

Eggplant Hasselback

Ingredients

1 Eggplant

1 cup Pizza Sauce

150 g Mozzarella Cheese, sliced

4 Cherry Tomatoes, sliced

4 tbsp. Parmesan Cheese, grated

1 tbsp. Olive Oil

1 tsp. Garlic, minced

½ tsp. Salt

¼ tsp. Black Pepper

Handful of fresh Basil Leaves

Preparation

- Preheat oven to 375F.

- Slice into the eggplant lengthwise, taking care not to cut all the way through.

- In a baking dish, spread pizza sauce on the bottom.

- Place eggplant on top of the sauce. Place slices of mozzarella, tomato and basil alternately between the eggplant slices.

- Sprinkle salt and pepper and drizzle with olive oil on top.

- Cover with aluminium foil and bake for 50 minutes.

- When eggplant is tender, remove foil and sprinkle parmesan on top.

- Broil for 5 minutes until the top is golden.

- Serve immediately.

Cashew Cream Stuffed Strawberries

Ingredients

2 cups Fresh Strawberries

1 cup Raw Cashews (soaked overnight)

1 tbsp. Maple Syrup

¼ cup Cream Cheese

1 tsp. Lime Juice

¼ cup 2% Milk

Preparation

- Drain the cashews of all the excess water. Place them in the food processor.

- Add lime juice and milk. Pulse until a grainy mixture is formed.

- Add water a little at a time, and continue to pulse until a smooth cream is formed.

- Transfer to a bowl.

- Cut off the tops of the strawberries and make a small hollow in the centre.

- Fill with the cashew cream neatly.

- Top with a small spoonful of cream cheese.

- Chill thoroughly and serve.

Egg White Scramble with Spinach and Tomato

Ingredients

4 Egg Whites

1 cup Fresh Spinach

6 Grape Tomatoes, halved

2 tbsp. Half and Half

2 tbsp. Parmesan Cheese

1 tbsp. Olive Oil

¼ tsp. Salt

½ tsp. Black Pepper

Preparation

- Heat olive oil in a non-stick skillet. Add the spinach and grape tomatoes. Cook for 2 minutes.

- Whisk the egg whites with half and half, salt and pepper.

- Pour the egg mixture into the skillet.

- Cook over medium heat. Allow the edges of the egg mixture to pull away from the skillet before lifting and folding the egg mixture so the uncooked eggs flow to the centre.

- Cook for 2 to 3 more minutes or until the egg whites are cooked through but still fluffy and soft.

- Sprinkle parmesan cheese on top and serve.

Avocado Cucumber Chickpea Salad

Ingredients

1 can (19 oz.) Chickpeas, drained and rinsed

1 Cucumber, diced

1 Avocado, diced

½ cup Feta Cheese

4 Green Onions, diced

1 tsp. Lemon Juice

1 tsp. Lime Juice

2 tbsp. Olive Oil

Salt and Pepper, to taste

¼ cup Parsley, chopped

Preparation

- In a large salad bowl, combine chickpeas, cucumber, avocado, green onions and feta cheese.
- Add the lemon and lime juice to the salad. Drizzle with olive oil and sprinkle salt and pepper.
- Toss well until well combined. Garnish with parsley.
- Serve fresh.

Caprese Style Portobellos

Ingredients

2 large Portobello Mushrooms

2 fresh Mozzarella Balls, sliced

2 tbsp. Olive Oil

2 tbsp. Balsamic Vinegar

1 tbsp. Red Wine

¼ cup Cherry Tomatoes, sliced

¼ cup Mozzarella Cheese

¼ cup Fresh Basil

2 cloves of Garlic, minced

Salt, to taste

Pepper, to taste

Preparation

- oven to grill setting on high.

- Cut off the stems of the mushrooms and wash and dry thoroughly.

- Mix olive oil with garlic and brush this mixture on the bottom of the mushroom. Place them brushed side down on a sheet pan.

- Brush the inside of the mushrooms with garlic olive oil as well.

- Fill the mushrooms with mozzarella and tomato slices. Season with salt and black pepper.

- Grill in the oven for 7-8 minutes or until the cheese has melted to a golden colour.

- In the meanwhile, combine red wine and balsamic vinegar in a small saucepan. Bring to a boil on high heat then simmer on low heat until thickened.

- Top the grilled mushrooms with the balsamic glaze and serve.

Tuscan Skillet Chicken

Ingredients

1 lb. Boneless Skinless Chicken Breast, sliced

2 tbsp. Olive Oil

1 can Crushed Tomatoes

1/8 cup Black Olives, pitted and sliced

¼ cup Sun Dried Tomatoes

¼ cup Chopped Onions

¼ cup Parmesan Cheese

1 tsp. Garlic, minced

1 tsp. Oregano

¼ tsp. Thyme

¼ tsp. Salt

¼ tsp. Black Pepper

Preparation

- Heat olive oil in a skillet and add onions. Sauté until soft.

- Add garlic and stir for 1-2 minutes.

- Add the boneless chicken and cook on both sides until it turns slightly brown.

- Transfer chicken to a plate. Add crushed tomatoes to the skillet and cook on medium heat.

- Add sun dried tomatoes and olives along with oregano, thyme, salt and pepper. Add parmesan cheese as well.

- Place chicken back into the skillet. Spoon sauce over the chicken.

- Cover and cook for 5 minutes on low heat.

- Serve.

Goats Cheese and Pistachio Stuffed Figs

Ingredients

 4 Fresh Figs

 2 oz. Goat Cheese

 1/8 cup Crushed Pistachios

 2 tsp. Honey

Preparation

- Preheat oven on grill setting.
- Cut figs into half lengthwise. Lightly press goat cheese into the centre on each fig.
- Sprinkle pistachios on top.
- Grill for about 5 minutes.
- Drizzle with honey. Serve warm.

Crumbly Berry Breakfast Bake

Ingredients

 1 cup Blueberries

 1 cup Fresh Strawberries, halved

 1 cup Raw Walnuts

 ¼ cup Almond Meal

 1 tsp. Maple Syrup

 ½ tsp. Cinnamon

 ¼ cup Rolled Oats

Preparation

- Preheat oven to 350F and spray a baking dish with non-stick spray.

- Pulse walnuts with almond meal and oats. Add cinnamon to the mixture.

- Layer the berries in the baking dish and toss with maple syrup.

- Generously spread the crumble mixture on top of the berries.

- Cover the dish with aluminium foil and bake for 10 minutes.

- Remove the foil and bake for another 10 minutes until the crumble is brown and crisp.

- Remove from oven and allow to cool. Serve with a dollop of Greek yogurt.

Crispy Parmesan Chicken with Vegetables

Ingredients

2 Boneless, Skinless Chicken Breasts

½ cup Grated Parmesan Cheese

1 medium Zucchini, sliced

1 medium Carrot, sliced

1 cup Green Beans

1 tsp. Garlic, crushed

2 tbsp. Olive Oil

½ tsp. Garlic Powder

¼ tsp. Salt

½ tsp. Paprika Powder

Preparation

- Preheat oven to 400F and line a sheet pan with parchment paper.

- Rub garlic onto the chicken and place in the sheet pan. Toss the vegetables with salt, paprika and garlic powder.

- Add to the pan along with chicken.

- Drizzle olive oil on top of the chicken and vegetables.

- Place the pan in the oven. Bake for 30-40 minutes, flipping chicken breasts halfway through.

- Sprinkle parmesan cheese on top of the chicken and broil for 3-4 minutes.

- Serve immediately

Herb Roasted Red Potatoes

Ingredients

1 lb. Red Skinned Potatoes

1 small Onion, chopped

1 tsp. Oregano

1 tsp. Dried Basil

1 tsp. Fresh Parsley

2 tbsp. Extra Virgin Olive Oil

½ tsp. Garlic Powder

¼ tsp. Salt

½ tsp. Black Pepper

Preparation

- Preheat oven to 400F. Line a baking sheet with parchment paper.

- Cut potatoes into wedges.

- Toss the potatoes with onion, oregano, basil, olive oil, salt, pepper and garlic powder.

- Transfer potatoes to the sheet pan.

- Roast for 30-40 minutes, turning occasionally until potatoes are tender and crisp.

- Serve hot.

Garlic Lemon Salmon

Ingredients

2 Skinless Salmon Fillets

1½ tbsp. Lemon Juice

2 tbsp. Olive Oil

4 Cloves of Garlic, crushed

2 tbsp. Fresh Parsley, chopped

2-3 Lemon Slices

Salt, to taste

Pepper, to taste

Preparation

- Dry the salmon fillets using paper towels.

- Mix lemon juice with salt and pepper. Rub this mixture generously onto the fillets.

- Heat olive oil in a non-stick pan. Press the salmon flesh side down into the hot pan.

- Sear for 3-4 minutes without trying to flip.

- Flip and sear the other side for 2 minutes.

- Add the garlic and parsley, drizzling with additional olive oil.

- Cook for an additional 1-2 minutes.

- Transfer to serving plates and garnish with parsley. Serve immediately.

Apricot Energy Bites

Ingredients

¼ cup Raw Almonds

½ cup Dried Apricots

1 tbsp. Unsweetened Shredded Coconut

1 tsp. Chia Seeds

¼ tsp. Vanilla Essence

½ tsp. Ground Cinnamon

Preparation

- Place almond in a food processor and pulse until roughly chopped.

- Add dried apricots, coconut, chia seeds, vanilla essence and ground cinnamon.

- Continue to pulse until chopped and mixed well.

- Take 1 teaspoon at a time and shape into balls.

- Refrigerate for at least an hour before serving.

Bonus Instant Pot Recipes

Instant Pot Chicken in Red Wine Sauce

Ingredients

> 4 Skinless Chicken Thighs
>
> ¾ cup Red Wine
>
> ½ cup Button Mushrooms
>
> 4 tbsp. Chicken Stock
>
> 2 tbsp. Olive Oil
>
> 2 Garlic Cloves, minced
>
> 1 tbsp. Tomato Paste
>
> ½ tsp. Dried Thyme
>
> ½ tsp. Corn Starch
>
> ¼ tsp. Salt
>
> ½ tsp. Black Pepper

Preparation

- Dry chicken thighs thoroughly on paper towels.
- Using the Sauté function of the Instant Pot, heat oil and add chicken thighs.
- Cook until golden, about 7-8 minutes.
- Transfer chicken to a plate and set aside.

- Add wine in the Instant Pot and stir to scrape the bits from the bottom.

- Add garlic, tomato paste, thyme along with salt and pepper. Stir to combine and add the chicken thighs back to the Pot.

- Cook on high pressure for 20 minutes.

- Release pressure manually. Add button mushrooms.

- Mix chicken broth with corn starch.

- Turn on Sauté function of the Instant Pot. Add the broth to the chicken while constantly stirring until the sauce has turned glossy and slightly thickened.

- Serve with mashed potatoes or on its own.

Instant Pot Margherita Casserole

Ingredients

1 cup Crushed Tomatoes

1 lb. Ground Chicken

½ cup Green Bell Pepper, sliced

¼ cup Black Olives, pitted and sliced

¼ cup Mozzarella Cheese

¼ cup Cheddar Cheese

2 Cloves of Garlic

1 tbsp. Olive Oil

1 tsp. Oregano

¼ tsp. Onion Powder

¼ tsp. Salt

¼ tsp. Black Pepper

Preparation

- Turn Instant Pot on Sauté option. Add olive oil and garlic.

- Once hot, add ground chicken and cook thoroughly. Season chicken with salt and pepper. Add onion powder as well.

- Transfer to a bowl and clean out the Instant Pot.

- Take a medium sized pyrex dish. Layer in the order of crushed tomatoes, ground chicken, bell peppers, olives, cheddar cheese and mozzarella cheese until 3-4 layers are formed.

- Sprinkle oregano on top. Cover the dish with aluminium foil.

- Add 2 cups of water in the Instant Pot and place trivet inside.

- Place the dish on the trivet.

- Cook on high pressure for 20 minutes. Release steam naturally.

- When pressure is released, remove lid of the Instant Pot and take out the dish.

- Remove the foil. Allow to cool for about 5 minutes before serving.

Mediterranean Hummus Recipe

Ingredients

1 cup dried chickpeas

1 tbsp baking soda

1/2 cup raw tahini / sesame paste

2 garlic cloves

1 lemon - juice only

1/2 tsp cumin

2 tbsp olive oil

salt and pepper to taste

Preparation

- Wash chickpeas, until water runs clean

- Soak chickpeas overnight, with baking soda

- Wash well, then drain the chickpeas

- Add chickpeas to a large pot of boiling water, bring to boil and simmer until the chickpeas are tender (about 90-120 minutes)

- Drain chickpeas, reserving the cooking water

- Blend cooked chickpeas, garlic, lemon juice, cumin, olive oil and seasoning in a blender or food processor. Add some of the cooking water, until hummus is the desired texture.

Ratatouille (4 servings)

Ingredients

3 red peppers, deseeded and chopped into chunks

250g courgettes, chopped into chunks

2 aubergines, sliced

2 tbsp. olive oil

2 red onions, sliced

2 garlic cloves

500g ripe tomatoes, chopped into chunks or 1 400g tin of chopped tomatoes

Sprig of fresh thyme

1 tbsp balsamic vinegar

Salt and pepper, to season

Preparation

- Heat olive oil in a saucepan and add peppers, courgettes and aubergine. Fry until softened and golden at the edges. Drain and spoon into a bowl.
- Add the onions and fry, until soft and sweet
- Add the garlic and fry for a few seconds
- Add the cooked vegetables and the tomatoes to the pan, together with the balsamic vinegar, salt and pepper
- Cover pan and simmer for 40 minutes, until the liquid has reduced
- Serve with crusty bread

Here's your final recipe, and it's my personal favourite, not least because it include an entire bottle of wine!

Cook in your slow cooker, for a sublime flavor, that you'll find you can eat almost every week.

Coq au Vin (Chicken in Wine) for 4 people

Ingredients

40g butter

6-8 pieces of chicken, leg or thigh

150g pancetta

2 onions

1 carrot, chopped

150g chestnut mushrooms, cut in half

2 tbsp plain flour

2 cloves garlic

A bottle of red wine (or add less wine, and replace balance with good chicken stock)

Bouquet garni

salt and pepper, to taste

Potatoes

Preparation

- Melt the butter in a saucepan. Add the chicken and brown the skin. Remove chicken from the pan and add to slow cooker or casserole dish.

- Add the pancetta, onions, carrot and mushrooms.   Fry gently, until onions are softened and sweet

- Add the flour and the garlic, stir until the flour is mixed well in with the vegetables

- Transfer vegetables to slow cooker or casserole dish

- Add the wine, together with bouquet garni, salt and pepper.

- Cook in the oven at 180C, for at least an hour, or in the slow cooker on low for 7-8 hours.

- Serve with boiled or mashed potatoes

9

AFTERWORD

You've heard how the Mediterranean is a diet unlike any other - it's a diet that's about more than just your food, it's about a more relaxed, fulfilling lifestyle.

You've learnt something about the science behind the diet, and all the many health benefits that are attributed to it.

You've discovered some of the so-called secrets of the diet, that you can start applying in your life this week.

And you've got the 14-day Mediterranean diet menu plan, together with 70 recipes you can start using today.

You have everything you need to start making the changes you want to see in your life, starting today.

I wish you all the best, as you make a start on the journey to a new healthier you, today!

Lisa Scott

LISA SCOTT

10

ONE MORE THING

If you've enjoyed this book, or found it helpful, please consider leaving a review.

Other books by Lisa Scott:

21 Day Keto Diet and Intermittent Fasting For Rapid Weight Loss - this book will tell you:

- the health benefits the Ketogenic diet

- how to fire up your metabolism for maximum weight loss

- the exact meals, contained in our 21 Day Menu Plan

- the results you can expect in 21 days

- how to keep the weight off with Intermittent Fasting

So many diets work for a short while, but then you pile all the weight back on.

Not this one - the Keto diet will help you lose weight fast and the Intermittent Fasting plan will help you maintain your weight. And you can see results in just 21 days!

If you'd like to start applying the principles of mindfulness to your life, why not try one of the following books.

Guided Meditation : for Anxiety, Stress Relief and a Quiet Mind - this guided meditation leads you through a full body relaxation, followed by a gentle guided meditation on the shores of a seashore, with the sounds of the waves lapping at the beach. This meditation will help you to: calm your mind, find relief from anxiety, relieve stress through mindfulness and find inner peace.

Mindfulness and Meditation for Beginners by Jen Carter - meditation is so much more than mantras and yoga. It's an ancient spiritual discipline, practiced by world religions for thousands of years. Research has shown that it's far more than just 'hippie' nonsense. In fact, it's been shown to have positive benefits for both our physical and mental wellbeing, reducing stress and combating depression and insomnia.

The power of mindfulness and meditation can help you clear your mind of unhelpful thoughts, control your stress and improve your sleep. Download this book to learn proven techniques for reducing the stress and anxiety in your life today.

CPSIA information can be obtained
at www.ICGtesting.com
Printed in the USA
LVHW060735270720
661604LV00016B/988